IN VITRO FERTILIZATION COMES TO AMERICA

Memoir of a Medical Breakthrough

Howard W. Jones, Jr., M.D.

Jamestowne Bookworks, Williamsburg, Virginia

D1205280

Howard W. Jones, Jr., M.D. is Professor Emeritus at Eastern
Virginia Medical School and the Johns Hopkins University

Jamestowne Bookworks, Williamsburg, Virginia
© 2014 by Jamestowne Bookworks
All Rights Reserved. Published 2014

ISBN 978-0-9897199-3-3 (print edition)
ISBN 978-0-9897199-4-0 (digital)

In vitro Fertilization Comes to America by Howard W. Jones, Jr.
Autobiographical history/memoir
Pioneering procedures in reproductive medicine
Medical ethics and law
Glossary

Jamestowne Bookworks LLC
107 Paddock Lane
Williamsburg, VA 23188

Front cover: The Drs. Jones with newborn Elizabeth Carr

IN VITRO FERTILIZATION COMES TO AMERICA

This book is dedicated to the team responsible for America's first IVF pregnancy

Mason Andrews

Georgeanna Seegar Jones

Anibal Acosta

Jairo Garcia

Lucinda Veeck Gosden

Edward Wortham

Bruce Sandow

Jeannine Witmyer

George Wright

Margaret Whitfield

Deborah Perry

Doris Gentilini

Debra Jones

And to my superb administrative assistant since 1979—
Nancy Garcia

Author Biography

Howard W. Jones, Jr., was born December 30, 1910 in Baltimore, Maryland. He received a Bachelor of Arts degree (*cum laude*) from Amherst College in 1931 and his M.D. from the Johns Hopkins University School of Medicine in 1935. He was a member of the staff of the Department of Gynecology and Obstetrics at Johns Hopkins until his mandatory retirement at age 65.

Besides responsibilities for patient care and medical education, Dr. Jones is and always has been a prolific author and editor. He held key positions in the development of ethical standards for reproductive technologies in the United States. He is a past Chairman of the Ethics Committee on Reproductive Technology for the American Society for Reproductive Medicine. Dr. Jones and his late wife, Dr. Georgeanna Jones, were the only American gynecologists invited by the Vatican to participate on a panel to advise Pope John Paul II concerning assisted reproduction.

Dr. Jones' early training and experience were in gynecological cancer. He was then involved in describing the precursors to the common type of cancer of the cervix which enabled early detection with the Pap smear and other technologies which substantially reduced the death rate from that disease. One of his patients was Henrietta Lacks whose cancer cells, known as

"HeLa Cells," proved to be immortal, and they continue to be of immense importance in basic and applied science.

While at Johns Hopkins, he became involved in reconstructive surgery of the internal and external genitalia of individuals affected by disorders of sexual development. He was instrumental in performing sex reassignment surgery for transsexual patients.

Following retirement from Johns Hopkins in 1978, Drs. Howard and Georgeanna Jones moved to Virginia to accept faculty positions at the Eastern Virginia Medical School in Norfolk. In that new institution they were challenged to establish an *in vitro* fertilization program, which successfully delivered the first American IVF baby—Elizabeth Jordan Carr—on December 28, 1981.

Table of Contents

Author Biography vi

Foreword by Elizabeth Jordan Carr Comeau xi

Preface xv

Acknowledgements xx

Publisher's Note xxii

    RISING TIDE OF DISCOVERY 1

    GOODBYE HOPKINS, HELLO NORFOLK 13

    NORFOLK 21

    TRIALS AND TRIBULATIONS .39

    IVF BEGINS IN AMERICA 55

    BREAKTHROUGH 75

    A SUIT FOR LIBEL 95

    IN THE VATICAN CITY 101

    THE QUESTION OF PERSONHOOD 135

    POSTSCRIPT FOR IVF 141

Glossary 151

Bibliography of Howard and Georgeanna Jones 157

Foreword by
Elizabeth Jordan Carr Comeau

I own a heart-shaped sterling silver necklace with the number "1" on one side and my initials on the other. I only wear it on special occasions as a mini good-luck charm or when I go to Virginia to visit Dr. Howard Jones, the driving force behind bringing IVF to the United States. The necklace is a kind of silent reminder of my roots, and a precious souvenir of the work that went into my birth: from mastering the science to presenting a case for IVF at The Vatican. This book is a glimpse into those endeavors by the man who led the charge—my doctor.

Growing up, I knew Dr. Howard and his wife, Georgeanna, were the doctors who made IVF technology in the United States possible, but I never appreciated what that meant until I was older. To me, Dr. Howard was and always has been part of my family. He signs my Christmas and birthday cards, "Grandad Jones," every year.

The first time I realized I was not like everyone else was when I watched the NOVA documentary of my birth—*A Daughter for Judy*. For all intents and purposes, it is my only "home movie," although it went through months of professional filming, editing, and post-production.

The experience of watching it was not, however, like

popping in a home-made DVD movie that makes you feel nostalgic for years gone by. Instead, I remember it felt like watching history unfold. I was just days old in the film, and the one making history.

I had seen the film only once before when I sat watching it seated between Drs. Howard and Georgeanna Jones, my legs dangling from the chair as the lights dimmed. We were not alone in the viewing room, but I recall that it felt like just the doctors and I were there. My parents did not attend. I know now it was because they could not think of better people to explain my conception than those two, determined, brilliant minds who had perfected the procedure. Throughout the documentary, I listened to the movie narrator, but paid special attention when Drs. Howard and Georgeanna explained what a Petri dish was, and when a doctor was performing a complicated task.

They explained, "The mother's egg and father's sperm are transferred to a Petri dish where they meet to divide and form an embryo which is put back into the mother's womb until the baby is born." They made it sound so simple, and it is how I explain my birth today.

There was no talk of how the Vatican published a document condemning In-Vitro, nor any mention of why I was born in Virginia rather than in Massachusetts, where my parents were living at the time. Nor did they say what would have happened if I had not been born a healthy baby. To my doctors and parents, it was a triumph that an infertile couple was able to have a child of their own, something they had all but ruled out after years of failed attempts. "There you are," I remember Dr. Georgeanna saying. "A beautiful little girl."

I never told my parents, but that was the day I realized the courage of that pioneering team of doctors. And it was when I realized that all the media attention I had gotten my entire life was misplaced, because I did nothing. I was just born! It was my doctors and parents who were special.

When I was ten, I got to meet and hold IVF baby numbers 1,000 and 1,001. They were twins, and symbols of how far the technology had advanced in just a short decade. I remember their parents telling me, "without you and your parents, our babies wouldn't be here."

But, in turn, without Drs. Howard and Georgeanna Jones at the helm in Norfolk, Virginia, I simply wouldn't be here.

Preface

This is a story of a medical program in Norfolk, Virginia, which resulted in the birth of the first IVF baby in the Americas and led to a revolution in the care of patients with infertility. The program was born in controversy, and might never have succeeded except for a remarkable series of chance events, encounters, and opportunities.

The first of those began long before we ever assembled our team and while my wife, Georgeanna Seegar Jones, and I were still on the faculty of Johns Hopkins Medical School. It was the arrival of Robert Edwards, a young Cambridge scientist who had been creating waves in his home country for daring to suggest that patients with blocked fallopian tubes could be helped to conceive children if their babies were conceived in a Petri dish.

Although undoubtedly the most daring and imaginative person in our story, who won the Nobel Prize for Physiology and Medicine shortly before he died in 2013, he was certainly not the only remarkable contributor to the breakthrough in infertility that afflicts so many and for which doctors down the ages have been almost helpless.

As books go, this is a short one, but I have endeavored to condense as much of this history for professionals, patients, and readers with a lay-interest in medicine so that they can understand that progress in any great venture is most likely when there is a convergence between the people fitted for the tasks and the circumstances and resources they need to succeed. The seeds of this story may have been sown in a great medical center (Johns Hopkins University), but they took root in most unlikely soil, a brand-new medical school in a corner of eastern Virginia.

If I told the story as a series of triumphant strides towards the goal, it would be a travesty of the record. How many worthwhile ends have ever been achieved without cost and sacrifice? The troubles that stalked Edwards and his colleagues across the Atlantic also visited us. That there are several million IVF babies in the world today is proof enough that the public has opened its arms to a controversial technology, because it has brought great happiness to so many. Some of the original arguments continue down to this day, creating a schism in society based, in my view, on an erroneous if perhaps well-meaning belief that personhood begins at fertilization. Despite our ability to manipulate and control human eggs and sperm using technology, conception remains, and always will be, one of the deepest mysteries commanding our respect. In this view, we are surely on the same wavelength as our erstwhile opponents who believed that IVF procedures are inimical to God's will.

The saddest part of writing this down is to remember that so many of the pioneers have gone—Bob Edwards, Patrick Steptoe, Jean Purdy, M.C. Chang, Ian Johnston, Carl Wood, and my beloved Georgeanna. And those of us who were young then are now getting on in age. As I look back to around 1930 in my student days at Amherst College,

Massachusetts, I recall my English professor was urging us in words that would become immortal, to take the "road not taken." We did.

Howard W. Jones, Jr.
Norfolk, Virginia
September 2014

Two roads diverged in a yellow wood,
And sorry I could not travel both
And be one traveler, long I stood
And looked down one as far as I could
To where it bent in the undergrowth;

Then took the other, as just as fair,
And having perhaps the better claim,
Because it was grassy and wanted wear;
Though as for that, the passing there
Had worn them really about the same,

And both that morning equally lay
In leaves no step had trodden black.
Oh, I kept the first for another Day!
Yet knowing how way leads on to way,
I doubted if I should ever come back.

I shall be telling this with a sign
Somewhere ages and ages hence:
Two roads diverged in a wood, and I—
I took the one less traveled by,
And that has made all the difference.

—Robert Frost

Acknowledgements

I wish to acknowledge the foresight of the late Mason Andrews, M.D., who was a founder of the Eastern Virginia Medical School and its first Chairman of the Department of Obstetrics and Gynecology. His support of our endeavors was prodigious, and without his encouragement the breakthrough in clinical IVF in America would have happened elsewhere and later.

The entrepreneurial courage of Glenn Mitchell, then Chief Executive Officer of Norfolk General Hospital, was also pivotal. He agreed to accommodate the program and provide support for our experimental and clinical investigations that became foundations for new and controversial reproductive technologies. The wisdom and counsel of Robert Nusbaum, LL.B. was critical in times of our greatest harassment.

Without the dedication and enthusiasm of the founding team of physicians, embryologists, nurses, and support staff, the story of IVF in America would have been different. I salute Georgeanna Jones, Anibal Acosta, Jairo Garcia, Lucinda Veeck Gosden, Edward Wortham, Bruce Sandow, Jeannine Witmyer, George Wright, Jr., Doris Gentilini, Deborah Perry, Margaret Whitfield, Nancy Garcia, Debra Jones, and Linda Lynch.

If our first patients had not been brave enough to try unproven procedures, our work would have foundered at the beginning. We would have been cast back to animal studies of dubious relevance, and a medical revolution in America would have been postponed.

In preparing this history, I thank Sabine Andrews (widow of Dr. Mason Andrews) for reviewing parts of the script.

It has also been my good fortune to have this book published by Jamestowne Bookworks. Dr. Roger Gosden has used his intimate knowledge of the field and his sagacity along with endless hours to make this book far more understandable and readable, especially to those not familiar with IVF history. And then there is Dr. Lucinda Veeck Gosden, a major player in this narrative. She corrected minor points, confirmed dates, and inserted arresting anecdotes that greatly improved the story. I lack adequate words to acknowledge my good fortune in having Roger and Lucinda once again as colleagues.

Parts of chapter 1 are based on, *Birthplace of a Breakthrough*, by Howard W. Jones, Jr., published by Hopkins Medicine (Johns Hopkins Medicine Publications, Fall 2013). Sections of chapter 9 have been adapted from chapters 3 and 4 in, *Personhood Revisited: Reproductive Technology, Bioethics, Religion and the Law*, by Howard W. Jones, Jr. (Langdon Street Press, Minneapolis, MN, 2013).

Publisher's Note

When Howard W. Jones, Jr., M.D. asked if this book could be published by Jamestowne Bookworks I was more than delighted: I thought it was a wonderful privilege and opportunity. There were three reasons for my enthusiasm.

As an elder statesman of American medicine, a memoir of his role as a medical pioneer ought to be important. It took talent, courage, and diplomacy to succeed in launching IVF for patients in this country. This is no ordinary story of medical progress, because it required a rare combination of circumstances, skills and people, and his team had to confront discouraging opposition for years. That they succeeded so well is told by the numbers of people who use the technology today and regard it as conventional practice and wisdom. We have added at the end of the book a complete bibliography of the works of the author and his equally distinguished late wife and collaborator, Georgeanna Seegar Jones, M.D., as perhaps the only public source representing their vast and long professional endeavors.

The second reason for wanting to publish this book is my personal connection with the author. I first met the Drs. Jones at a scientific workshop at Bourn Hall, Cambridge, exactly thirty years ago in November 1984. They flew to England from Virginia to contribute to round table discussion about novel reproductive technologies, which was hosted by my late mentor, Bob Edwards. I remember the other participants were excited to meet the American pioneers. I had read papers about their IVF program in medical journals, but I would not meet one of their co-authors (Lucinda Veeck) until nearly twenty years later when I joined the Jones Institute, and afterwards married her. Lucinda and I continue to be in regular contact with Dr. Howard since we live in the same state once more.

Lastly, I welcome *In Vitro Fertilization Comes to America* because we published the life of the New York surgeon-naturalist, Robert Morris, last year. It is particularly fitting to follow with a story told by another remarkable innovator and thinker.

This book is not aimed specifically at readers of medical history; I believe that many patients, doctors, and students will enjoy Dr. Howard's personal account of a medical breakthrough.

Roger G. Gosden, Ph.D. (*Cantab*), D.Sc. (*Edin*)
Jamestowne Bookworks LLC, Williamsburg, VA
http://www.jamestownebookworks.com

1
RISING TIDE OF DISCOVERY

This story begins in Cambridge in 1963 with a young British physiologist, Bob Edwards (1925-2013), a few years before we started working together at Johns Hopkins University. He joined the Marshall Laboratory under Sir Alan Parkes in the University's Department of Physiology as a Ford Foundation Fellow and would become the Nobel Prize-winning, Sir Robert Edwards. Bob rose to the rank of full professor in a position specially created for him, and he continued to work in that department until his retirement.

Much earlier in his career when he was trying to develop a contraceptive vaccine with the Medical Research Council in London, he became intrigued with news of embryo research in the laboratory of M.C. Chang (1908-1991) at the Worcester Foundation in Massachusetts. Bob never wavered in his fascination for embryos, even when his job description required working on other problems.

Chang was a distinguished Chinese-American scientist who collaborated with Gregory Pincus in the development of the first birth control pill, but by 1959 his attention focused on promoting fertility rather than inhibiting it. He used rabbits to provide the first indubitable evidence of *in vitro* fertilization (IVF) of a mammalian egg, although there were earlier, controversial claims of priority. Building on the discoveries of the French biologist, Charles Thibault (1919-2003), Chang observed two pronuclei were present in rabbit oocytes (eggs) after inseminating them in culture: one contained the genetic endowment of the father and the other of the mother. He needed to prove to critics that fertilization had occurred, rather than parthenogenetic activation which results in unfertilized eggs because there is no involvement of a sperm. He avoided ambiguity by creating embryos from the oocytes of albino rabbits fertilized with sperm from black rabbits, which he transferred into the uterine horns of albino surrogates. The litters should be black if they inherited the paternal genome during fertilization—they were!

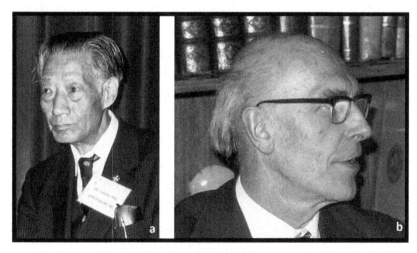

(a) M.C. Chang in Norfolk, Virginia,
(b) Charles Thibault (1978).

Chang emphasized that *in vitro* fertilization could also be confirmed at the time of conception provided that, in addition to the two pronuclei, there was a sperm tail embedded in the oocyte's cytoplasm (the jelly-like substance filling the cell). Thibault had been endeavoring to achieve fertilization in a variety of species in the 1950s and 1960s, but he only succeeded in showing that two pronuclei were present in his published work. Without proof of a sperm tail, the scientific community thought his evidence was not sufficiently robust to prove *in vitro* fertilization had occurred. This standard of proof later became important for us as well.

Towards the end of 1978 I was invited to the Collège de France in Paris to visit the laboratory of Alfred Jost. He was the leading expert in the developmental biology of the female and male generative tracts, which was relevant in my earlier surgical career but at that time I crossed the ocean for a different purpose. My visit occurred soon after I had moved to Norfolk, Virginia, and we were then in the process of building a clinical IVF program. When Jost heard this news, he invited Thibault to join us for an afternoon at the college to discuss progress he was making with *in vitro* fertilization in animals. Thibault was optimistic about success with IVF in humans since it had already been proven in laboratory animals. The question of needing a sperm tail in the cytoplasm to confirm that fertilization had occurred was raised, just as it had been over a decade earlier when Bob and I were making our first endeavors with human fertilization outside the body.

After Bob moved to Cambridge in 1963, he was eager to follow up Chang's success by attempting *in vitro* fertilization in mice. His model species was decided by the availability of a mouse colony in the Marshall Laboratory, and he had done graduate and postdoctoral research on mouse genetics in Edinburgh under Conrad Waddington. He became increasingly obsessed with the notion that IVF could be—and should be—applied to humans, but development of the technology would need a supply of human oocytes from clinical sources. He contacted every obstetrician and gynecologist in the Cambridge phone book, but none offered to help him.

He therefore expanded his search for clinical collaborators to London where he received an encouraging reply from Molly Rose, the obstetrician who had delivered two of Bob's daughters while he was working at the Medical Research Council in Mill Hill. She supplied him with small ovarian biopsies on five separate occasions over a period of about two years. For each specimen, he had to drive a round trip of over a hundred miles to London, which meant sacrificing the whole day. Details of how he maintained the specimens during the journey and how the oocytes were extracted in the laboratory are covered by the dust of time, although he explained those efforts to us in considerable detail when he first came to Johns Hopkins in 1965.

We know that he generally managed to tease out three to five oocytes from each specimen. Not all—or perhaps none—were mature cells, and so it is not surprising that when they were incubated with sperm, fertilization never occurred. There was also a question of whether fresh sperm would be mature enough for successful fertilization. Independently in the early 1950s, Chang and "Bunny" Austin (who succeeded Parkes as head of the Marshall Lab) showed that sperm in animals needed to be exposed to the environment of the female reproductive tract for a few hours before they became competent to participate in fertilization. It was not known if this phenomenon, which they called "capacitation," applied in humans as well, or if it could be achieved outside the body in culture medium. It is quite understandable that Bob became terribly frustrated by limited research material and discouraging results.

His wife, Ruth Fowler, was one of his research collaborators since their graduate days together in Edinburgh, so she understood his vexation. She suggested that he contact Victor McKusick (1921-2008), who was then Chief of Medical Genetics at the Johns Hopkins School of Medicine, to ask whether it would be possible for him to obtain human oocytes for research. The letter Bob wrote to Victor was forwarded to me, although I did not realize at the time that it would open a new research path for the rest of my career. I was then a member of the Department of Gynecology and Chief of the Cryogenetics Laboratory at Hopkins. As I did not know Bob, I replied through Victor saying that I thought it was entirely possible to supply oocytes. I was confident in making this offer because at that time a standard therapy for treating polycystic ovarian disease (PCO) was wedge resection of the ovaries, and this was and remains a relatively common endocrine disorder in women.

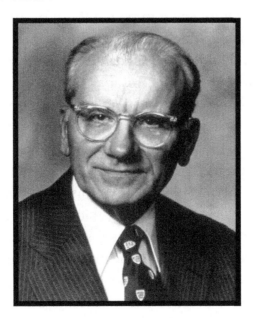

Victor McKusick.

We were doing one or two resections per week, and it seemed perfectly feasible to give Bob a portion from each wedge. A normal human ovary weighs about eight grams, but a polycystic ovary averages about 30 grams, from which we usually resected about a third. It seemed to me that if we gave Bob half a wedge, he could have about five grams of tissue: the remainder was required for pathological examination.

This was the protocol we adopted when Bob arrived in Baltimore as a visiting research fellow in July 1965. He succeeded in teasing 8 to 12 oocytes from each half wedge. Although most of the oocytes came from women with PCO, a few whole ovaries became available from patients who required complete removal of one or both ovaries for a variety of reasons. Bob transferred his small harvest of oocytes to culture medium in a Petri dish where he hoped they would mature overnight by resuming meiosis, which halves their chromosome complement in preparation for fertilization. At first he cautiously added to the medium samples of the fluid that had bathed the oocyte inside the ovarian follicle, but this was found to be unnecessary. He also discovered that it was unnecessary to add any specific hormones to trigger maturation, which was usually complete after overnight culture. Among his most important observations was the fact that oocytes matured "spontaneously," as they did in animals, and this became the subject of his first published paper from Hopkins. It was much later that other researchers uncovered the cytoplasmic proteins responsible for controlling oocyte maturation, including the master regulator known as the anaphase-promoting complex/cyclosome.

Besides these studies, Bob was anxious to understand how to capacitate sperm for fertilization. Capacitation was a rather neglected topic when he was experimenting with specimens from London, and only became relevant after oocytes could be matured *in vitro*. Back in 1951, when Chang and Austin discovered that freshly ejaculated sperm were incapable of fertilizing oocytes in animals, they realized that sperm need to sojourn for 8-10 hours in the fallopian tubes before they become competent. Bob had many discussions with us about how to ensure capacitation under experimental conditions, preferably *in vitro* because transferring sperm to a human fallopian tube or uterus and retrieving them again for fertilization after capacitation was experimentally onerous and ethically dubious. He suggested that spare pieces of human genital tissue from surgery might help if they are co-incubated with sperm in a culture dish. This was theoretically plausible, as well as practicable, because at the time it was thought that the tissue secreted substances affecting sperm as they ascend to the site of fertilization, near the end of the fallopian tube. It was my role to furnish the samples.

The sperm were washed in saline by what we now call the "swim-up technique" to avoid transferring blood and to remove any dead sperm. After hopefully capacitating the sperm, we added them to cultures of fresh oocytes from ovarian wedges. The oocytes were most precious, and only numbered 56 in total.

The results are still interesting all these years later. After 24 hours in culture, there were seven oocytes that had degenerated, and another 17 still possessed a germinal vesicle nucleus, implying that they had not progressed to metaphase II of meiosis when normal fertilization occurs. Another 26 oocytes had matured completely as evidenced by a first polar body, but none of these were fertilized. However, three others had two beautiful pronuclei, presumably carrying both the male and female genetic contributions, and one had four pronuclei. We wondered if these were not pronuclei what else could they could be? Since in those days we believed there were vital secretions from the female tract, a saline wash was assumed to be inadequate for capacitating sperm, and because sperm tails were never observed in eggs, the matter was closed with a shrug of the shoulders. In retrospect, however, we may indeed have been observing normal fertilization in a dish for the first time in history since we now know capacitation only requires the removal of certain molecules from the sperm surface, and this can be achieved simply by washing them. Moreover, there are continuing doubts whether, at least in humans, capacitation is actually required at all.

"Fertilization" of only three out of 56 oocytes might seem a poor result but, considering the cells had not been recovered from timed menstrual cycles and the majority was immature, it looks much more encouraging. The egg with four pronuclei was obviously abnormal, possibly because it had been penetrated by three sperm cells, or perhaps by two sperm if one of the sets of female chromosomes had not been excluded during meiosis. Eggs with three pronuclei remain relatively common today in clinical IVF and are discarded. They would create a chromosomally abnormal embryo which is inviable or might create a pathological "molar pregnancy."

We also tested the fertilizing ability of sperm that had swum through human cervical mucus collected from the middle of the menstrual cycle, since this is one of their milestones on the journey to the site of fertilization. Hoping that sperm exposed to the mucus would be capacitated, we mixed them with seven mature oocytes, but none developed pronuclei and were presumed to be unfertilized.

In another set of experiments we tested tissue from a fallopian tube that had been removed from a patient on the 17th day of her menstrual cycle, which was lucky because it was close to the normal time of ovulation and fertilization in the body. Epithelial cell scrapings were incubated in culture medium with 20 oocytes, 15 of which matured. Two oocytes each contained two pronuclei the next day but, since we could not confirm sperm tails in the cytoplasm by microscopic examination, we had to discount these cells from evidence of fertilization.

Such disappointments led us to attempt human sperm capacitation inside the uterus of rabbits. After varying lengths of incubation, the sperm were flushed into dishes containing 118 oocytes in all. Three oocytes later appeared to have pronuclei, but this could not be confirmed when they were fixed on glass slides for detailed examination.

We then turned to a primate model because there was a macaque monkey colony at Hopkins. One of our fellows, Ted Baramki who later became a faculty member in the department, joined the project in August while Bob Edwards was still with us. He had experience of working in the Cytogenetics Laboratory and was an early practitioner of amniocentesis, going on later to perform about 3,000 cases up to the year 2000. When five macaque monkeys became available for study, Ted helped us transfer 67 mature human oocytes plus large numbers of sperm to the fallopian tubes in a series of operations. There was never any risk of making human-monkey hybrids because human sperm cannot penetrate the outer membrane of a simian oocyte! This procedure later became well-known in human clinical practice as GIFT

(Gamete Intra-Fallopian Transfer), although it is seldom practiced today. At intervals of 12 to 18 hours after transfer, the animals were examined by hysterectomy with bilateral salpingectomy so that Bob could attempt to flush cells into a dish for microscopy. After so much effort, the results were bitterly disappointing because only two unfertilized oocytes were recovered. We still do not understand what happened to the gametes, although they evidently perish rather rapidly in monkeys. We learned a lesson that to be viable gametes must develop in the appropriate species and environment.

These experiments were published in the September 1966 issue of the *American Journal of Obstetrics and Gynecology* under the title, *Preliminary Attempts to Fertilize Human Oocytes Matured in vitro*, with Bob Edwards, Roger Donohue (technician), Ted Baramki, and myself as coauthors. We cautiously called our results "preliminary" because we only had the evidence of fertilization from pronuclei, yet it has turned out that a sperm tail in the cytoplasm is not needed as an absolute criterion for success. Two pronuclei are now generally accepted as evidence that fertilization has occurred, so we had in fact unknowingly succeeded in achieving the first fertilization of a human egg.

After returning to Cambridge, Bob must have sensed that our work at Hopkins was crucial for developing IVF as a beneficial procedure for patients with infertility because in his book, *A Matter of Life: The Story of a Medical Breakthrough* (1980), he wrote that he left Baltimore feeling "exultant" and his experiences had been "decisive."

That year, 1965, was "decisive" for me too because if circumstances had been different, I doubt that clinical IVF would have blossomed in America soon after our move from Baltimore to Norfolk in 1978.

It scarcely needs to be stated that on returning home to Cambridge, Bob continued striving towards his goal. In 1968, he began to collaborate with Patrick Steptoe (1913-1988), a senior British gynecologist who served patients in the town of Oldham, which is about a three hour drive north of Cambridge and not far from Manchester. It might appear strange that he did not have a clinical partner at one of the leading academic medical centers in Cambridge or Oxford or London, which were so much closer to his base, but most British gynecologists were wary, regarding him as a daring radical. His work was coming under increasing criticism from public figures and in the press. But Steptoe was his perfect partner because, despite training at St. George's Hospital, he was not a member of the London establishment and had a reputation for being his own man. More importantly, he was the national pioneer of laparoscopy, a minimally-invasive technique that Bob needed for harvesting oocytes from patients if a program offering IVF was ever to get off the ground. They established a clinical research laboratory in Oldham while Bob maintained basic research at Cambridge. Jean Purdy was the third member of their team, a nurse who was recruited by Bob to run what became their clinical embryology laboratory.

Except for Bob and Jean, other personnel in Cambridge were largely left in the dark about the progress being made, perhaps to protect junior researchers from involvement in a controversial research agenda. Indeed, such was the secrecy that many were unaware that a breakthrough had taken place until the announcement of Louise Brown's birth in Oldham on July 25, 1978. The public criticisms that the trio had endured for a decade were then turned upside down as their nation's newspapers celebrated Louise as, "The Baby of the Century!"

I am telling this story not only to give credit to Bob and Patrick for working out the details of a revolutionary medical technology, but also to show how tentatively IVF moved forward and to provide a background for its coming to America. And when it arrived, it was received with a mixture of pride, awe, and horror.

2

GOODBYE HOPKINS, HELLO NORFOLK

I shared an office in the Women's Clinic of the Johns Hopkins Hospital with my wife, Georgeanna, who was a pioneering reproductive endocrinologist. Along with other members of the staff, we saw our patients in offices nearby, which was a fine arrangement for many years. But as full-time faculty members of the University, our contracts required us to retire at the end of the academic year in which we reached 65 years of age. For me, this meant June 1976, and for Georgeanna two years later. We discussed various options for accommodating the gap, but never hit on a plan that seemed to be completely satisfactory.

Sometime during May of 1976, I received the expected retirement notice from the Dean's office, and that same day I had a telephone call from the hospital president. He understood that I was due to retire at the end of June, but since Georgeanna occupied the same office as I did—and we had a partners' desk—my departure would not release space that could be reallocated to other staff members if she continued working until the full retirement age. He assured me that the hospital would approve if I continued to use the office as before until that time.

Hence, we now had a plan which simplified things tremendously, and when 1978 rolled in, we consulted our own children for advice. They unanimously urged us to take retirement seriously and enjoy fishing in the Chesapeake Bay for which our busy careers had hitherto spared little time.

However, when others heard that we were leaving Hopkins, other opportunities were suddenly presented to us which threw us briefly into confusion again. We were invited to join the staff of a medical school in New Orleans, and another one in Philadelphia for a couple of years. There was also a call from Mason Andrews (1919-2006), a gynecologist we had known for many years and a Hopkins graduate like ourselves, who invited us to join the newly created Eastern Virginia Medical School (EVMS) in Norfolk. Mason was the first Chairman of its Department of Obstetrics and Gynecology, and at that time there were only two other members on his faculty. He told us that if we were to accept, it would be our role to start and organize a division of what we now call the subspecialty of reproductive medicine.

This was certainly the most interesting offer because it was a completely fresh challenge with the prospect of working with an old and much-respected friend and his wife, Sabine. We settled on this option enthusiastically and had to scramble to sell our Baltimore home and find a new one in Norfolk.

I have likened Mason Andrews to Sir Thomas More because he too was, "a man for all seasons." Besides his full-time career practicing gynecology in the City of Norfolk, he was the moving spirit behind the creation and development of EVMS. He believed that the institution could help to build medical services and education in an underserved corner of Virginia. He was also dedicated to civic affairs and had been a member of the City Council since 1974. The governance of Norfolk reflected its English origin, its council consisting of seven members from which the mayor was elected by a majority of four votes. It was a part-time job because the city manager took care of day-to-day affairs.

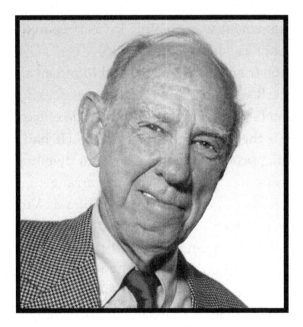

Mason C. Andrews: "a man for all seasons."

Somewhere around July 10, 1978, I received a call from Mason who told me that an election was coming up and he was assured of the four votes to become mayor. The dean of the medical school did not think it was appropriate for a chairman of a department to be the Mayor of Norfolk at the same time. It was lucky that I was well-acquainted with him because he suggested that if I was willing to accept the reins of chairman, Mason could be freed to become Mayor.

This was a turn of events I was not prepared for because I had been acting chairman at Hopkins for a while and was not particularly keen to continue in the same role after my "retirement." Besides, I was worried that I would be regarded as an unwelcome outsider by other members of the staff, none of whom I knew. When I expressed my reservations to Mason I did, however, leave a little loophole. I said that if no other arrangement was possible I was prepared stand in for him, but only as a last resort.

As a true friend, Mason tried and found an alternative arrangement. It was not status that he was seeking in a public appointment, but the opportunity that the office presented of launching a cherished hope for Norfolk. He had a vision of a new housing project to replace the slum dwellings. After our phone discussion, I learned that an arrangement had been made to create a special position for him as Vice-Mayor for city redevelopment so that he could continue to serve as a departmental chairman. I received this news with a sigh of relief since I could now refocus on our original plans.

Because houses were not selling briskly at that time in Baltimore, we decided to leave our furnishings behind and rent furniture for a new home in Norfolk until a sale went through. We were lucky because, at the very last minute, the house was sold and we hurriedly arranged shipping of the furniture we needed and disposal of the rest. The problem was that we did not yet have a home to move into!

Those were busy months for us; we had little spare time for the five-hour drive to Norfolk to hunt for houses. Georgeanna had looked at a couple of possibilities, but neither was exactly what we wanted, and I too had made a

search that ended in disappointment. But our discourage-
ment did not last long because Sabine Andrews called with
news of a house that was being advertised in her district. I
hurried to Norfolk where she picked me up at the airport to
drive me to Shirland Avenue where a realtor had left a notice
at the verge of number 7506.

It looked a perfect fit because the home promised not
only to comfortably accommodate the two of us but also
Asbury who had lived with us in Baltimore for many years
to help run the house and raise our family. There was a private apartment at the Shirland residence that fitted his needs
perfectly. Concerned that we might be scooped, I immediately bought the property knowing that Georgeanna would
approve when she saw it.

When the morning for our move rolled around on July
25, 1978, a large truck turned up outside our Baltimore
home, but it was 4:00 p.m. or even a little later before all
the furniture was loaded for the journey to Norfolk. We left
with Asbury around 5:00 p.m. in our old Ford station wagon
which was filled like a barge with precious possessions that
we could not trust to movers. After spending the night at a
motel in Bel Alton, Maryland, we made a rendezvous with
the truck the following day around 1:00 p.m at our new residence in Norfolk.

Unknown to us while we slept in Bel Alton, Louise
Brown was being delivered by Cesarean section by Patrick
Steptoe at Oldham, in the north of England. She was the first
child ever created by a new and exciting method of concep-
tion, IVF. We heard the news on the radio while driving to
Norfolk the next day.

That afternoon we were still busy moving in when at
about 3:00 p.m. the telephone rang for the first time in our

new dwelling. It was Julia Wallace, a newspaper reporter from the local morning newspaper. She explained she had already called Mason Andrews for a reaction to the sensational news in England which was blazing across the world. At the close of the interview he told her that we had worked with Bob Edwards. He urged her to call us. She arrived on our doorstep two hours later, and because we had not yet unloaded our chairs, we had to sit on packing boxes for the interview. We described to her what we knew of the process of *in vitro* fertilization, and why it was a wonderful breakthrough for childless couples.

As she was leaving, she cast a final question: "Could this be done in Norfolk?"

"Of course!" It was a light reply to what I thought was a flip question, and I never anticipated her next question.

"What would it take to do it here?" she asked.

"It would take some money."

The next day we read her article in the newspaper. She described what had been assimilated from the many reports about Louise Brown's birth and how she had been conceived in a laboratory Petri dish. At the end, she quoted me saying that this could be done in Norfolk, but that it would require money.

The very next day we received another unexpected phone call while we were still arranging our things. This time it was from a Norfolk patient who had been referred to Georgeanna by Mason Andrews when we were working in Baltimore. As a result of her treatment, she had gotten pregnant and even named her daughter "Georgia" after my wife. This kind lady said that until she saw the morning newspaper, she had not known we had moved to the Tidewater area. But her phone call was not just a cordial welcome to Norfolk; it was my throw-away remark about needing money to start an IVF program that prompted her to contact us. She asked something I have never been asked before or since, "How much do you need?"

We arranged to meet the woman and her husband at home two days later to discuss the offer they were making anonymously. Without their generous help, I don't know how we would have gotten started. Mason and Sabine Andrews joined us at the meeting, accompanied by Henry Clay Hofheimer, a well-known and highly-respected Norfolk businessman and chairman of the board of the EVMS Foundation. I was already familiar with his name because a neighbor in Baltimore encouraged me to meet him, and even wrote a letter of introduction. They had been together as members of the Federal Reserve Board when it met in Richmond. Henry Clay later became one of our most influential supporters. Any new clinical enterprise, however, especially one that is likely to stir controversy, is impossible without the support of your departmental chairman. In Mason Andrews we not only had someone on our side from the very beginning, but also an ardent enthusiast who was actively pushing us from behind. In time, he also lent a hand at a vital moment in our program.

3

NORFOLK

Within a week of moving to Norfolk, our plans had ballooned enormously. But the scope of creating an IVF program *de novo* and the trials ahead were still beyond comprehension.

Settled in my assigned office in the Medical Tower, I thought I should call Bob Edwards to congratulate him on the breakthrough of Louise Brown's birth. When I got through, he immediately recognized my voice even though it was well over a decade since we worked together. We had a stimulating conversation about the events leading up to her birth and the publicity surrounding it. He then explained that the contract of a consultant doctor in the British National Health Service required Patrick Steptoe to retire at age 65, which he had already reached. That was a serious interruption of their work at the very time when they were at last able to offer hope to patients who were clamoring for fertility treatment.

I told Bob that we were starting an IVF program in Norfolk and would be grateful for any help he could offer.

"Would it be possible," I asked, "for your assistant, Jean Purdy, to come to Norfolk to help get us started?"

Bob handed the phone to her in the room next to his office.

Jean said she would have to think about it, but on a follow-up call the next week she regretfully declined. Bob and Patrick were now planning to open a private clinic at Bourn Hall where she was urgently needed.

About all the technical advice I could get during those trans-Atlantic calls was Bob's advice to stick to the natural menstrual cycle because, in their experience, pregnancies failed every time they tried to stimulate ovaries with hormones. Undoubtedly, there were advantages of using such an approach: the timing of ovulation could be controlled, more oocytes would be available, and laboratory scheduling would be easier. Nevertheless, we heeded his advice. He did mention that they were using a standard culture medium for fertilization and embryos, but never provided any details on this crucial question. He wished us well, and that was that. We were on our own.

Since the procedure developed by the British team required a hospital environment, our first task was to recruit the support of the Norfolk General Hospital, which was then a free-standing hospital on the medical school campus. Its director, Glenn Mitchell, was a former administrator at Hopkins whom I already knew slightly, which helped when I approached him about starting an IVF program in his hospital.

I explained the medical and technical processes involved and what we would need: a dedicated operating room available at short notice around the clock, an adjacent embryology laboratory, and a recovery room where patients could rest without being disturbed by through-traffic. After a short discussion, Glenn replied that he knew of an unused room in the delivery suite which had never been occupied since it was built. There was an adjacent sterilization room which he thought might be converted into a small laboratory. And, lastly, an unused room nearby could very well be converted for sole use by patients recovering after procedures.

I was delighted and quite surprised that suitable facilities could be made available so easily, and without more ado. Moreover, he was prepared to provide any equipment that we needed in the operating room, as well as contribute towards incubators, microscopes, and anything else required in the laboratory. I felt blown-away by this generosity. In hindsight, I wondered if Glenn was hoping that we might eventually create a new medical service that could turn a handsome profit for the hospital. If that was indeed in mind, his investment turned out well.

Within a short period of around two weeks, we were busy converting the rooms into an O.R. and a laboratory. It was not long before the clinical protocols I had in mind were ready for execution.

Since we had decided to follow Bob's advice and collect oocytes during the natural cycle, we would monitor hormones on an outpatient basis to predict when ovulation was likely to occur. Each patient would be called for admission to the hospital about six hours before ovulation was expected, and since that could occur at any hour of the day or night it meant that the surgical and laboratory teams had to be available seven days a week and around the clock. After a patient's oocytes had been collected by laparoscopy she was transferred to the recovery room for a few hours, and depending on whether her eggs were fertilized and she had a transfer, she would then have a bed on the ward for a day or two.

The two founding members of our IVF team, Mason Andrews and myself, were already on the OB/GYN faculty at EVMS, and we needed to recruit others. Anibal Acosta was the first. He came to Johns Hopkins Hospital in 1959 to join Georgeanna's endocrine and infertility service. His girlfriend, Rosita, was still living in Córdoba, Argentina, and wanted to join him in Baltimore, but her family vehemently opposed their unmarried daughter moving to the USA, even though they knew Anibal quite well. The matter was resolved when they married, which was arranged over a telephone call between the two continents. Rosita settled down with him in Baltimore, and I recall their union was solemnized in a ceremony at which they could join hands this time.

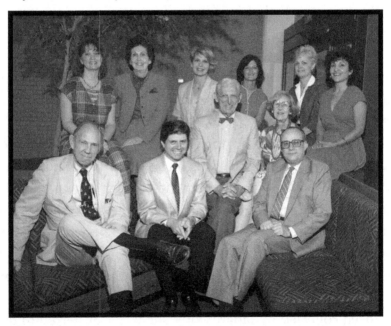

The original IVF team in Norfolk (listed left to right).
Front row: Mason Andrews, Jairo Garcia, Howard
Jones, Georgeanna Jones, Anibal Acosta. Back row:
Deborah Perry, Doris Gentilini, Lucinda Veeck, Linda
Lynch, Nancy Garcia, Margaret Whitfield.

Anibal became a clinical fellow in the department while Rosita was hired as a laboratory technician. He came with valuable experience gained while working with Georgeanna for measuring a gonadotropic hormone which gives advance warning of when ovulation will occur, and which determines, in turn, when patients are scheduled for laparoscopy. The assay method was originally based on rats. On the Acostas' return to Argentina after a couple of years in Baltimore, they carried four cages of inbred rats from the Hopkins colony on the airplane to start their own animal colony. In those days, scant attention was paid by airport security to carry-ons, even small livestock! We visited the couple on more than one occasion, and I was later honored by the University of Córdoba with an honorary degree of *Doctorate, Honoris Causa*.

Juan Peron was President of Argentina on-and-off from 1946 until his death in 1974, at which time he was succeeded by his third wife, Eva. Peron instituted a strict form of socialist government which was based on his studies of Italian and German politics before World War II and came to be known as Peronism. It was a rigid regime that stifled independent thinking, even in universities such as Córdoba where Anibal worked. By 1975, he and Rosita decided they needed more freedom to pursue their work, and hoped to return to the United States. That is how I received his inquiry.

There was no possibility of bringing him back to Hopkins because, although I was on the faculty, my retirement date loomed on the horizon. But I knew that Mason Andrews in Norfolk was assembling a new department at EVMS and was having trouble recruiting capable clinicians. After referring Anibal, he was in due course appointed as chief of service at the affiliated Catholic DePaul Hospital. One of his roles was to supervise resident staff at the Norfolk General Hospital who rotated through DePaul Hospital. Anibal was only the third full-time member of the OB/GYN faculty at that time.

He was eager to join our endeavor as soon as we started the IVF program at Norfolk General, and became a key member of the team. His training in the diagnosis and treatment of male infertility was particularly valuable because, although it was not uncommon in South America, it was much rarer in the United States for a gynecologist to oversee male infertility. He did, however, have some uncomfortable experiences from being affiliated with an IVF program while being based in a Catholic hospital, even though he himself had grown up in that denomination. The Church took its time in declaring an official attitude to the new assisted reproductive technologies (ARTs), but when *Donum Vitae* was published in 1987, its opposition was stated unambiguously (see Chapter 9). Anibal then felt the heat.

The Church adopted the position that if IVF caused abortions, it was inherently evil. These were not the kind of abortions one usually envisions of a fetus with an emerging human form attached to a placenta, but the loss of free-floating fertilized eggs which mostly perish as a microscopic ball of cells without implanting after transfer to the uterus. Sometimes they miscarry later on after more development. Since the Church recognized that personhood and ensoulment starts in the single cell after fertilization, it was adamantly opposed to IVF from the very beginning.

Anibal's position as chief of service at DePaul reached a crisis in 1980 from the conflict between his work and the Catholic doctrine the hospital adhered to. The spark was lighted by a nurse who reported to the administration that he had performed an artificial insemination procedure for a patient in his hospital office, which was certainly contrary to Catholic doctrine though routine practice in most institutions. He ultimately resigned from DePaul and moved into offices with the OB/GYN staff at EVMS where he contributed enormously to the IVF program because of his expertise in both male infertility and female endocrinology. In fact, in the following year, it was Anibal who aspirated the oocyte from Judy Carr's ovary that was fertilized in our lab and became the first IVF baby in the New World.

In the early 1970s, I was occasionally invited to South America to speak at OB/GYN conferences. As most meetings were in Spanish, I accepted on the condition that I could arrange for Anibal to be present as a simultaneous translator. One of those occasions was in Quito, Ecuador, in July of 1973. At the close of a session, I was approached by a young Colombian doctor who needed Anibal to help him with English. This was Jairo Garcia who had already met Georgeanna and was trying to arrange a fellowship at Johns Hopkins. We were both so impressed with Jairo's energy and enthusiasm that we wanted him to join the training program. After his application had been processed and approved in Baltimore, I wrote him with the good news. Unfortunately, he never received my letter because by the time of writing he had changed his address in Colombia, and the letter was never forwarded to a new one.

Sometime later he was accompanying his mother-in-law to our hospital where she was being admitted as a patient. On encountering Anibal in a corridor, Jairo asked him to relay to me the fact that he had not heard about his application. When I learned about the miscommunication, we finally managed to have him appointed as a fellow and he moved to Baltimore with his wife, Nora, in 1974 and stayed until 1976.

Some two years later at the end of 1978, as we were

struggling to organize the IVF program in Norfolk, it was obvious that we needed more hands. In one of those happy coincidences that helped us move forward, Jairo wrote to us from Colombia. The political situation there was very troubling and he inquired whether it might be possible to return to the States with his family to join our team.

Jerry Holman, who was medical dean at the time and an old friend from Hopkins, managed to find funding for Jairo to join us in April of the following year. Jairo proved to be a great addition as the fourth member of our medical team and possessed a flair for new techniques. In those early days, we wondered if shearing forces from the negative pressure needed to aspirate ovarian follicles might harm oocytes. Suction pressure created by drawing back the plunger of a large hand-operated syringe was neither well-controlled nor measurable. Jairo succeeded in fitting a measuring device and reassured us that we need not worry about damaging eggs. He stayed with us, becoming a full member of the clinical staff.

Coming from the same background as Anibal, he had to make some accommodation in his work to avoid violating Roman Catholic directives. In due time, Jairo and his wife Nora quietly resolved the issue, and he fully participated in the momentous transfer of the Carr embryo. Jairo returned to the Baltimore area in 1985 to establish a new IVF center, and twelve years later moved to Johns Hopkins Hospital to become director of its IVF program. He remains there today.

The last of the original five members of the medical staff was certainly not the least. My wife, Georgeanna Jones, had long been acknowledged as an international leader in the field of reproductive endocrinology and infertility. She began her career in June of 1939 when she was appointed by Richard TeLinde on the very day he was confirmed as the first chairman of a separate gynecology department at Hopkins. She became the director of an independent section of the department that specialized in infertility and hormone research. At the time she was only 26 years of age, and she kept that position for a stately tenure of 39 years until her forced retirement.

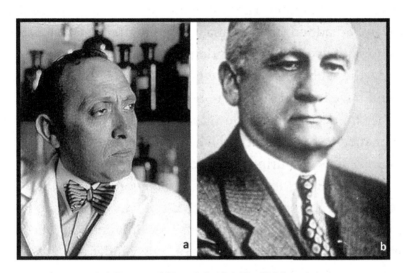

(a) Bernard Zondek, (b) Emil Novak.

As a medical student, Georgeanna proved that the placenta is the source of the pregnancy hormone that we now call human chorionic gonadotropin (hCG). The hormone had been discovered earlier by the German-Jewish endocrinologist, Bernhard Zondek, but he suspected that it originated in the pituitary gland.

Zondek, who had moved from Germany to Palestine because of Nazi persecution, made a visit to Hopkins in 1939 to see Emil Novak, who was the most distinguished gynecological pathologist of his day and a tireless author and editor. With the chairman of obstetrics, Nicholson Eastman, Novak had founded *The Obstetrical and Gynecological Survey*, and continued to make scientific contributions until his death in 1957 when Georgeanna and I took over the editorship for the next 27 years.

When Novak arranged a luncheon for Zondek at the Maryland Club in downtown Baltimore, it was a swanky club for businessmen that required the names of guests to be approved ahead of time. The club manager, surprised to see that Novak had added Georgeanna's name to the guest list, called him to politely deny her attendance. Women were not allowed inside the club. Novak replied that if she was barred they would have to meet elsewhere because it was most important for her to meet Zondek. He was the co-developer of the first pregnancy test (A-Z test) which was based on the discovery that injections of a urinary extract of hCG triggered ovulation in animals. The club relaxed its opposition so that the luncheon could go ahead as planned, but it was some years later until other women were admitted. This tidbit of scientific history is one of the stranger stories of how gender equality was slowly advanced and, in this instance, involved hormones and rats. Times have changed, they say, and the current president of the Maryland Club is a woman.

In addition to her expertise in treating endocrine pathology when a hormone deficiency causes infertility, Georgeanna always found time for research. In 1949, she was the first to describe the so-called "luteal phase defect" in which progesterone secretion ends too early to support conception, and two decades later she reported the ovarian insensitivity syndrome in which follicle-stimulating hormone (FSH) from the pituitary gland fails to promote ovarian follicle growth. Her earlier experience of inducing ovulation in anovulatory women with pituitary extracts of gonadotropic hormones and with the synthetic drug, clomiphene, before it became commercially available, was particularly valuable to us. In fact, she was ideally qualified for some of the most difficult challenges we would face in developing an IVF program.

It fell to me, with my surgical background, to take charge of the laparoscopic procedures for egg collection, which required adapting the techniques from general use. Unless I was successful at this stage, no oocytes would be collected for fertilization and, therefore, no embryos to transfer.

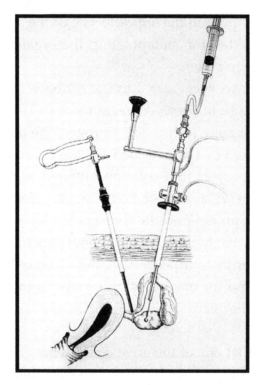

*In the early days, a laparoscope was used to
retrieve oocytes from follicles in the ovary.*

The Norfolk method of egg retrieval differed in certain details from the procedure used by Patrick Steptoe. He used a "needle plus three puncture technique." He first inflated the abdomen by inserting a needle through the umbilicus, using nitrogen rather than the usual carbon dioxide to maintain a more physiological pH for the oocyte. When the abdomen was sufficiently distended, a puncture wound was made for introducing the laparoscope. This allowed inspection of the viscera. In addition to this puncture wound, there were two more punctures in the lower abdomen, one on each side. One was used to insert the needle through which the egg was retrieved from the ovary using suction apparatus. Through the other puncture port on the opposite side of the abdomen, forceps were inserted for manipulating the organs so that the ovary was in good view.

In Norfolk, we were afraid to use nitrogen to distend the abdomen because in previous years there had been fatalities with the use of air, which is 80% nitrogen. We therefore used carbon dioxide, but compensated for the concern about pH by collecting oocytes in a solution buffered at pH 7.4. This seemed to work. A laparoscope with an offset lens enabled us to insert the aspirating needle through the laparoscope itself so we did not need to make an additional puncture in the lower abdomen for that purpose. Also, there was only one lower puncture wound for manipulating forceps to make sure that we could see the ovary.

I often muse that one of the great coincidences that helped to promote our program was that all five of us had spent parts of our careers at Johns Hopkins. I wonder if exposure to the unique academic chemistry of that institution had a role in preparing us for the challenges we faced together in Norfolk and helped to become a strong team. Mason, Georgeanna and I were medical students at Hopkins before World War II and received our residency training there. Although Anibal and

Jairo started their careers in South America, they became fellows working in our services there. Our common background gave us all an earnest and inquisitive outlook that we brought to medical care and training of others.

As the practice of IVF advanced, it became clear that the partnership between clinicians and clinical embryologists was critical for success. There are few, or perhaps no, specialties in which the balance and mutual respect between these halves of a medical service is more important. Consequently, it was vital to appoint the right people to lead the embryology lab, and it was a decision we pondered carefully.

We were already very familiar with collaborating with clinical laboratory scientists since our Hopkins days. In those days, I was involved with a cytogenetics lab headed by Jack Rary for my work on inter- and trans-sexualism. It became a very busy center with two full-time technicians and two or three fellows who rotated through. When we moved to Norfolk it became redundant because the work on intersexualism was transferred to two other departments, and the hospital decided it would no longer offer transsexual surgery. Hopkins' loss was our gain because it provided an opportunity to move unwanted equipment to Norfolk where it was needed. Moreover, Jack decided to move at the same time to become head of the cytogenetics lab at the Norfolk General Hospital.

Jack soon had the lab up and running and as the workload grew he needed to recruit someone to provide technical help. That person was Lucinda Veeck (later, Gosden), who had recently graduated with certification in medical technology. No one at that time in the United States, and hardly anyone in the world, had experience with IVF technology, but we knew that expertise for culturing human cells in the cytogenetics lab was a strong baseline with which to start. We asked Jack if he could provide assistance to make our embryology lab functional and, after asking a host of questions, he and Lucinda agreed.

The entire team spent considerable time discussing the medical, surgical, and laboratory equipment we needed. Compromises had to be made to keep within a tight budget, and in the end it was Jack and Lucinda who took charge of sending out orders and testing equipment after it arrived. Increasingly, these matters became Lucinda's responsibility, and at some point before our first IVF pregnancy Jack asked to be relieved of duties which were hard to balance with his primary responsibility for cytogenetics. Lucinda, however, stayed on.

We could not open the embryology laboratory for clinical cases until we were granted a Certificate of Need in 1979 (Chapter 4). We did, however, have a start-up budget from the hospital and public donations, although they barely covered the costs of basic equipment, of which an incubator, two microscopes, and a laminar flow hood were most important and expensive. With such a meager inventory it hardly mattered that the lab was tiny (just 6x15 feet), but it sufficed for our purposes and we were thankful for it.

The American Fertility Society (now the American Society for Reproductive Medicine) is the national body that represents professionals working in the field of fertility treatment. Soon after IVF appeared as a novel therapy, the Society laid down requirements for running a clinical embryology lab, which included a clause stating that the laboratory director should have an earned Ph.D. degree in a relevant discipline. Accordingly, Ed Wortham, who had a doctorate from Old Dominion University, was recruited to the post. This seemed a good plan because Old Dominion was already part of our network and where Anibal Acosta was doing semen examinations that could not be done at DePaul Hospital. Sometime later, sperm banking was added to the male fertility services based at Old Dominion.

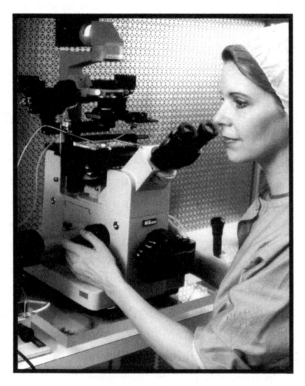

Lucinda Veeck.

Lucinda was always involved in the day-to-day running of embryology and was officially appointed as its director when Ed Wortham left to take a position in Oklahoma in 1982. She was, and is, a detail-oriented person and a meticulous worker, and these characteristics are fundamental for a successful IVF program. It can be stated without reservation that the care of eggs and embryos *in vitro* is no light task! In those early days, Jeannine Witmyer, from Old Dominion University, and Bruce

Sandow, from EVMS, worked alongside Lucinda in the lab. Before long, Lucinda was being called as a conference speaker around the world and as a consultant for new treatment centers. Her reputation spread not only from news of our clinical success but as a teacher and author of books that continue to adorn the bookshelves of embryologists worldwide.

We already had support staff in position for the general clinical service. There were nurses and secretaries, and my administrative assistant, Nancy Garcia, and nurse, Doris Gentilini who were major stalwarts. As the program grew and patients flooded in, we needed to hire more staff.

We were concurrently deluged with requests from professionals from far and wide who sought clinical or laboratory training or both in our center. Our first embryology fellows were both from Italy: Vera Montacuti and Giulietta Micara. Vera traveled to Norfolk along with one of our first international clinical fellows, Anna Ferraretti. Giulietta was sent by Professor Carenza of the University of Rome "La Sapienza," and she stayed for a year, returning home to start her own very competent IVF program. After a visit to Bari, Italy, yet another Italian fellow, Simonetta Simonetti, was sent by her supervisor, Professor Bettocchi, but when he died unexpectedly and his successor was disinterested in IVF, she stayed on with us for seven years. She became a highly competent embryologist and a trainer herself.

Of the foreign clinical fellows who worked and studied in Norfolk, Themis Mantzavinos from Athens was the first, and he overlapped with Anna Ferraretti from Bologna. Over the years, literally hundreds of clinical and laboratory fellows rotated through our doors. Since accommodation of visitors who wanted to witness laparoscopic retrievals in the O.R. was limited, we used a closed-circuit television, which was still novel

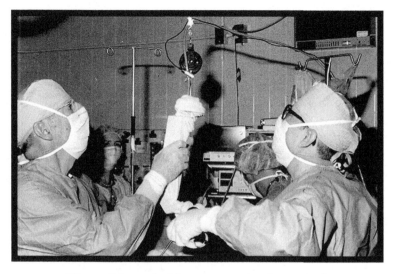

Howard Jones holds a camera to photograph
an operative procedure.

then. There was a TV camera the size of a brick and almost as heavy that we attached to a stand overlooking the operating table for transmitting both images and commentary to an adjacent room accommodating about ten more people. During these sessions, the eagerness of our team was apparent—each time an oocyte was recovered successfully, a round of gentle cheers and soft clapping erupted in the O.R., usually led by Georgeanna. She always made herself available for holding patients' hands during procedures for moral support, and I have been told that this tender picture is one of the most enduring memories for many of our fellows and visitors. Visitors looked forward to question-and-answer sessions after retrievals and transfers. Everyone was eager to learn the Norfolk way of doing IVF, and this tide of approval seemed ironic because, before the program was rolled out, we had to face serious opposition and an unexpected administrative hurdle.

4

TRIALS AND TRIBULATIONS

At the beginning of 1979, there was a dramatic event which, in hindsight, was a harbinger of things to come.

One night early in January, a taxi driver who was passing the Norfolk Medical Tower that housed our offices noticed flames erupting from a window about halfway up the building. He called the fire department. The fire was in Mason Andrews' office which had just been refurbished. His desk was completely destroyed and he lost patient files, lecture slides, personal mementos, and family photos which had hung on the walls. Nothing in his office was recoverable. Investigators from the Fire Department who questioned him and other members of staff eventually concluded that it was caused by arson, but the person(s) responsible was never identified. Suspicion fell on a nightwatch man, who was never seen again.

Georgeanna and I were out of town at that time and returned to find our offices were damaged too, but never imagined that within a few weeks we would be engulfed in flames of controversy.

A little earlier, while we were busy organizing the program, the chief hospital administrator, Glenn Mitchell, telephoned to let me know that the regulations then in force required us to have a "Certificate of Need" before a new clinical service could be opened. Any delay was unwelcome, but he assured us that because we were launching a completely new program within the United States, the hospital would have no trouble getting a green light to proceed. He explained it was a routine matter that might even be granted administratively, which is to say without a public hearing. He would take care of the application so I would not be put to any trouble. These reassurances put me at ease, but not for long.

Much to the surprise of all, a number of people turned out for the review meeting to protest against our application. That rarely happened, if ever. They had evidently been alerted by the local newspaper which routinely published notices of such meetings. I was not present, but afterwards I heard that the protests ranged from pseudo-theological arguments that we were playing God, to ethical objections that *in vitro* fertilization would cause abortions. The abortion argument has lasted longest, and occasionally raises its head even today.

About a month after the hearing, the Commissioner of Health for Virginia, James Henle, sent an official response to the Norfolk General Hospital because our application was made in the name of the hospital and not in our own names. The following is extracted from his letter.

> *Based upon that review and the need to resolve questions and issues regarding the scope of the project, your request for a Certificate of Need under the Administrative Review Process has been denied for the following reasons:*
>
> *The proposed project has statewide implications and*

should be reviewed by the Virginia Statewide Health Coordinating Council (SHCC). The Standard Review Process provides for the SHCC to review and formulate a recommendation concerning the statewide need for a proposed project under the Certificate of Need Program.

The In Vitro Fertilization Laboratory project appears to be only one component of a comprehensive infertility treatment program. The Standard Review process will allow for a review of all (emphasis added) components of the comprehensive infertility treatment program.

It will be necessary, if the project is to be pursued, to complete and submit an application which will be reviewed in accord with the standard review process identified in Section 6.00 of the Virginia Medical Care Facilities Certificate of Public Need Rules and Regulations.

The necessary Certificate of Need application forms for filing under the standard review process are enclosed.

Glenn Mitchell called to break the devastating news that our request had been turned down. We had never expected that outcome. However, he told us not to worry and that he would follow up the commissioner's suggestion, if I agreed.

We had the strong impression that the commissioner was influenced by recent passions stirred up by our proposals. Perhaps we had been too sanguine since we were, after all, living in a conservative corner of the state; only a few miles away in Virginia Beach sat the Christian Broadcasting Network and Regent University founded by Pat Robertson. The commissioner's letter did not, however, make any mention of the protests. His denial of approval was issued on a technicality, namely that our application for a Certificate of Need only referred to the embryology lab rather than being a more inclusive petition for a "comprehensive infertility treatment program." Mr. Henle had only asked for us to be compliant with the rules for a standard review. We had to admit that we had made a bureaucratic gaffe, and hopefully one that could easily be rectified.

Before reapplying, I thought we should take the precaution of getting the boards of both the hospital and the medical school on our side. I therefore asked if I could appear before them to explain details of what we were proposing. In taking this course, there was a risk of running into complications since I did not know all the members of those boards. Thankfully, we received unanimous approval to go ahead with our plans, and many members urged us forward.

I conveyed the news to Glenn, who made a fresh application for review at a public hearing. The meeting was scheduled for Halloween Day in 1979, with opening comments presented at 2:00 p.m. It lasted a full six hours. The publicity generated by the earlier protests had encouraged much wider public interest, not only in bringing out more sympathizers, but drawing newspaper reporters and TV crews from the NBC, ABC, and CBS networks.

Unbeknownst to us, we had plenty of our own allies. Newton Miller, who later became an OB/GYN practitioner in Norfolk, organized some of his fellow medical students as well as house staff to attend the hearing, which was held at the Norfolk Public Health Department building. His efforts succeeded so well that most seats were filled in the auditorium an hour ahead of time. When busloads of protestors began arriving, they found there were no more seats available inside, and officers from the Fire Department would not allow standing in the aisles. The crowd gathering outside was frustrated, although emotions cooled when seats became available after medical students had to leave for classes and duties. The hearing got underway after a slightly delayed start.

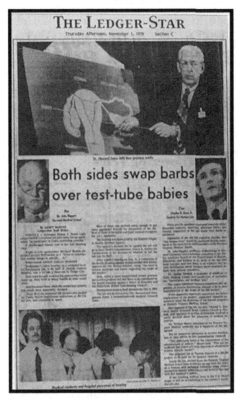

Newspapers provided extensive coverage of the hearing in Norfolk to consider a Certificate of Need for IVF.

We were prepared for an organized opposition and an articulate plea for embryos to be granted "rights-to-life." We had invited several distinguished doctors and scientists from outside to speak in defense of *in vitro* fertilization. Roy Parker was then president of the American College of Obstetricians and Gynecologists and chairman of OB/GYN at Duke University, and John Biggers was a Harvard Professor of Physiology and an old friend from Hopkins days. We also had on our side the Right Reverend Heath Light, an Episcopal bishop and former rector in Norfolk who was familiar with our plans. Lastly, Lawrence Foreman was a well-respected Rabbi of the Ohef Sholom Temple in Norfolk, and he spoke eloquently in support of our program. On the other hand, and most surprising to us, incredible claims were made by protestors that *in vitro* fertilization would surely promote incest, human-animal hybrids, and other bizarre scenarios which were both shocking and unbelievable.

The protests did not cease after the hearing but continued right up to the time when the decision was announced. There were articles in the media almost daily and we received a great deal of correspondence. Among the hostile ones was a letter from Charles Dean who was then president of the Tidewater chapter of the Virginia Society for Human Life. It was circulated to a number of individuals and organizations, and I reproduce it here in full because he expresses a point view that is seldom heard today.

> *We write to you as fellow members of the human family, members who seek to make the voice of reason prevail against the so-called Test Tube Baby Program at Eastern Virginia Medical School, and more particularly against the granting of a Certificate of Need for an 'In Vitro Fertilization Laboratory' proposed for Norfolk General Hospital, an indispensable element for the project's viability.*
>
> *As you know, Dr. Kenley denied the first application which was submitted under the Administrative Review Process because he felt the implications of 'In Vitro Fertilization' mandated a more full consideration and review.*

Indeed they do. The hospital's second application, submitted under the Standard Review Process, will soon be before you.

Having attended the public hearing October 31st and listened to the arguments pro and con from about eighty scheduled speakers, and having sifted through more than 2,000 pages of testimony to the federal Ethics Advisory Board on this subject, the root question has come into brilliant focus. Have the proponents of the Norfolk project embarked upon this seemingly compassionate undertaking after a thorough and adequate study of this terribly complicated subject with its many and multifaceted ramifications? Regrettably, but most assuredly, the answer is NO.

The Ethics Advisory Board of the Department of Health, Education, and Welfare is the primary repository of information on this subject. Although it had been empaneled in early 1978 to consider a funding application for In Vitro Fertilization without embryo transfer, the scope of its enquiry was broadened to include almost all aspects of the subject following the birth of Louise Brown in England July 25, 1978. That board was not even close to the conclusion of its investigation and had not even begun its deliberations for a decision when a six year old medical school in Norfolk, Virginia captured national and international headlines by announcing it would have the first so-called Test Tube Baby Clinic in the United States. We wondered at the wisdom of that when it occurred, but we did not actively oppose the project until the Ethics Advisory Board had concluded the hearings, made its deliberations, and made its decision which was most inconclusive.

The Board's decision defined ethical acceptability as possibly falling into one of three classifications. It said that it was

not finding this kind of activity to be 'Ethically Mandatory.'
Neither did it find it to be 'Clearly Ethically Right.' It found
it to be 'Ethically defensible though still legitimately contro-
verted.' The Board went on to say that it "wishes to make
clear that in reaching a decision as to 'acceptability,' it is not
finding that the ethical considerations against such research
are insubstantial."

Although we would like to cover in detail the many and
varied moral, medical and legal arguments which should
bring about a denial of the application, since they are ex-
plored in depth in other testimony which will be in your
hands, we will for the purpose of this letter explore one gen-
eral area. As a scientific matter, it is accepted that a proper
foundation must be laid for anything which will stand the
test of time. A proper foundation for this particular project
has indisputably NOT been laid in that the risks to mother,
and more particularly to prospective child, have not yet been
determined. One of the most respected doctors in America
who testified before the Ethics Advisory Board is Leon R.
Kass, M.D., Ph.D. of the University of Chicago. In his ex-
pert testimony to the board, he stated, "The attempt to gen-
erate a child with the aid of In Vitro Fertilization constitutes
an experiment on that child." Concerning the risks of such
experimentation, Dr. Kass said, "... caution is the posture
of responsibility toward such prospective children. I would
agree with Doctors Luigi Mastroianni, Benjamin Brackett,
and Robert Short that the risks for humans have not been
sufficiently assessed, in large part because the risks in ani-
mals have been so poorly assessed (due to small numbers of
such births and to the absence of any prospective study to
identify and evaluate deviations from the norm)."

Proponents of the local project say they have all the data they need from the study of 'animal husbandry.' They also say it would be expensive to conduct clinical research on sub-human primates, and they say such research would take too much time which they do not wish to spend. Obviously, the study of 'animal husbandry' (largely farm animals which are bred for short-term slaughter) is a grossly inadequate scientific base to justify I.V.F. experiments on human beings. Once again, please note Dr. Kass' remarks above. The second and third reasons, we believe, are the real reasons why the project is being pushed so hard by the proponents, and we find that extremely interesting in light of remarks made recently by Professor Jerome Lejeune. Professor Lejeune is the Chairman of Genetics at the University of Paris and is one of the most respected medical scientists in the world, having discovered the chromosomal anomaly responsible for Mongolism [sic] (ed., Down syndrome), and having been awarded just about every major honor which could be bestowed upon a man of medicine. At a seminar on In Vitro Fertilization of which he was a co-lecturer with Sir William Liley (the so-called Father of Fetology) in Canada recently, Professor Lejeune said,

"TO THE BEST OF MY KNOWLEDGE, I CANNOT SEE ANY RESULT WE COULD OBTAIN BY EXTRA-CORPOREAL FERTILIZATION (I.V.F.) IN MAN WHICH WE COULD NOT OBTAIN JUST AS WELL DOING THE SAME THING IN CHIPANZEES [SIC], OR MONKEYS IF YOU WISH. NOW, YOU HAVE TO ASK YOURSELF THE QUESTION WHY PEOPLE WHO WANT TO EXPERIMENT ON A HIGHLY COMPLICATED LIVING SYSTEM LIKE PRIMATES CHOOSE TO DO IT ON MAN AND NOT ON

CHIPANZEES [SIC]? THE REASON IS VERY SIMPLE AND VERY DRAMATIC. WE HAVE BEEN TOLD FOR CENTURIES THAT HUMAN LIFE WAS PRICELESS. NOW, I CAN TELL YOU, IT HAS NO PRICE AT ALL. IT COSTS A LOT TO HAVE A CHIPANZEE [SIC] FEMALE, TO HAVE A TINY (I.V.F.) CHIPANZEE [SIC] BEING GROWING, AND TO PUT IT BACK IN THE WOMB OF THE CHIPANZEE [SIC] MOTHER. YOU HAVE TO PAY A LOT FOR THAT. BUT THE TINY HUMAN BEING HAS NO PRICE NOWADAYS. YOU CAN KILL IT. IT DOES NOT COST ANYTHING TO MANIPULATE IT BECAUSE IT HAS BEEN ABANDONED ENTIRELY, EVEN BY THE PARENTS. SO, WE ARE FACED WITH THE HORRIBLE FACT THAT IF THOSE EXPERIMENTS ARE PROPOSED IN MAN (I.V.F.), IT IS NOT BECAUSE THEY CANNOT BE MADE IN ANIMALS, BUT BECAUSE IT WOULD COST A LOT IN ANIMALS, AND IT DOES NOT COST A DOLLAR TO DO IT ON HUMAN BEINGS. THAT IS THE VERY TRUTH YOU HAVE GOT KNOW."

What Professor Lejeune has said is a profound commentary on contemporary society. The question for us is whether we are going to continue down the same road, whether those in positions of authority such as yourself will by their decisions begin to turn our society back in the direction of the highest ideals of true civilization, one of the hallmarks of which is the protection of all human life.

Your decision in this matter can make a difference, and we urge you to consider thoughtfully what is at stake, and voice your opposition to the application.

Charles Dean was not a lone voice. The *Virginian Pilot*, a Norfolk newspaper published an interview with the Catholic bishop, Walter Sullivan, who appealed to his diocese and beyond to "have the courage to stand up against the proposed 'test tube' baby laboratory at Norfolk General Hospital." He claimed that defective human embryos would be discarded and abnormal fetuses would be aborted in the process. Sullivan contended that adoption would be a more Christian response to childlessness, because "[adoption] places love for an existing child over the needs of parents for a blood heir."

Despite all the hostile attention, the Norfolk General Hospital received a letter approving our application from its Executive Director, Paul Boynton.

On September 20, 1979, the EVHSA Project Review Committee, on behalf of the Eastern Virginia Health Systems Agency, acted upon the Administrative Review request submitted by Norfolk General Hospital to establish a laboratory in support of the In Vitro Fertilization Program.

I am pleased to inform you that the Committee approved the following recommendations, which have been forwarded to the State Health Commissioner.

That the Administrative Review request by Norfolk General Hospital to establish a genetics laboratory in support of the In Vitro Fertilization Program be approved for the following reasons:

The costs associated with the proposal are minimal.

The proposal warrants special consideration as a research project designed to meet national needs.

The proposal is consistent with the recommendations of the DHEW Ethics Board.

The proposal has been approved by the local Human Experimentation Committee as required by DHEW.

The project violates no law or canon of bio-medical ethics.

Since no other such service appears to exist nationally, accessibility to and availability of such service will be increased for women of Eastern Virginia and women residing elsewhere in America. Thus, American women and particularly Eastern Virginia women, who otherwise would be unable to have children, will be able to receive a service which possibly will enable them to have children.

The Eastern Virginia Health Systems Agency sincerely appreciates your cooperation during the review process.

Some six weeks after this approval for the Certificate of Need, the staff of the Norfolk General Hospital passed the following resolution.

The staff finds that patients will experience serious problems in terms of availability and accessibility in obtaining this service in the absence of the proposed program for the following reasons:

There are no known existing programs in the United States; thus, the Vital Initiation of Pregnancy Program [VIP Program] would allow availability and accessibility of a presently non-existing service.

At least 280,000 women in the United States who are unable to have their own children because of oviduct dysfunction and who would not be assisted by the existing surgical alternatives would be candidates for this type of program.

In view of #2 and the number of inquiries (over 2,000)

received by the applicant, the program could reasonably yield the projected utilization of 50 patients the first year.

This program would make available to women in Eastern Virginia and women residing elsewhere in America, who otherwise would be unable to have children, a service which possibly will enable them to conceive and bear their own children.

Disapproval of this program may constitute denial of a fundamental right and may, thus, be legally indefensible.

However, there were some dissenters, and among them the anesthesia group that served the hospital. In February of 1980 when we were about to begin clinical trials, I received a letter from their office manager.

In view of our present shortage of anesthesiologists and prior commitments for their services, we regret we will be unable to supply coverage for any in vitro fertilization proce-dures. We feel that we are presently unable to provide cover-age for these cases without defaulting on our commitments for both scheduled and emergency coverage.

At first sight, this letter seemed to be a road-block for our clinical trial which was scheduled to start in the next few weeks. Fortunately, however, two anesthetists in the group approached me privately to express a willingness to work with us, and assured us that this offer was made with the full knowledge of their colleagues. Quincy Ayscue, one of the pair, would become the anesthetist for Judy Carr when she had a Cesarean section for the birth of Elizabeth.

Before we received the Certificate of Need, the hospital

works department had already started to construct our embryology laboratory. But when it appeared that we might have difficulty getting approval, the lab was sealed with tape, as was the delivery room next door which was destined to become the egg retrieval room. The closing off of these rooms was so thorough that it would not be obvious to anyone that any construction had yet taken place, which could have been embarrassing.

The publicity generated by the hearings had the unintended consequence of drawing attention from far beyond the Hampton Roads community. Inquiries poured in from childless patients who, after having had no success through their own doctors, pinned their increasingly desperate hopes on IVF in our program. This attention caught us by surprise because we had planned to start gradually, only accepting patients at first from our own practice whom we thought had the best chances of success. With the gathering pace of clinical activity, we decided it was prudent to present our plans to the Patient Review Committee at our own hospital. The modern equivalent is the Institutional Review Board (IRB), which consists of a group of professionals and lay-people who have the ethical responsibility of protecting the rights and interests of research subjects. Since IVF was certainly regarded as an experimental treatment, it was apropos to review the risks and benefits for patients we were recruiting for treatment. The review process also required us to prepare information sheets for patients and a consent form for them to sign after they had read the documents and had been appropriately counseled.

To be accepted, couples had to be generally healthy and the women younger than 35 years of age with regular menstrual cycles and a normal uterus. The male partner was expected to have a normal sperm count. These criteria excluded a lot of patients, but in time advances in reproductive technology enabled women to have children through IVF who were much older, had anovulatory cycles, or even lacked a uterus. And from the 1990s, a man possessing very few sperm could be helped to become a genetic parent using a new technique (ICSI), which avoided the need for donor insemination.

An additional requirement then (but no longer) was that women have a bilateral salpingectomy (removal of both fallopian tubes), although that was not mentioned on the form. The rationale was owing to an early criticism of Edwards and Steptoe's program that pregnancies attributed to IVF might have, in fact, been conceived naturally. The absence of fallopian tubes also avoided the risk of ectopic pregnancy, an unfortunate situation that had occurred in one of the first British patients to become pregnant after IVF.

We knew we would be under intense scrutiny as the program unfolded, and so we decided only to accept married couples in the beginning. Today, the treatment of unmarried couples and single women is so common that it hardly draws comment, but public attitudes were much more conservative then. Somewhat surprisingly, it was this decision that worried the committee most of all. A minority of members pointed out that if this requirement stood, it would exclude some of them or members of their families from becoming candidates for treatment. Because of this, we subsequently changed our criteria to include couples in a "stable relationship," however that might be defined. Indeed, it was ultimately defined on an individual basis by drawing on clinical experience.

As responsible and caring physicians, we resolved to waive our professional fees for patients until such time as we had succeeded in producing a live birth. The hospital and medical school could not be so generous, needing to levy a modest charge which was calculated on an out-of-pocket basis, but which excluded our salaries from the formula. Thus, patients were expected to pay a small fee for hospital accommodation and drugs and most were well-satisfied with this policy. Moreover, they were not deterred by knowledge that they would be undergoing an experimental procedure which was uncomfortable and time-consuming with no guarantee of success. We marveled at their willingness to undergo repeated treatment and invest their hopes in the program, which certainly drove us even harder to help them succeed.

5

IVF BEGINS IN AMERICA

Since the time when Bob Edwards came to work with us in 1965, we kept regularly in touch with him. When he was visiting the States, he would often stop in Baltimore for a day or two to spend time with us in the hospital or at home. I fondly remember he was particularly interested in the history of the American Civil War, and on one of those trips we drove to the Gettysburg National Military Park for a day. As Bob usually traveled here unaccompanied, we never had an opportunity to meet his clinical partner, Patrick Steptoe. After the birth of Louise Brown, we were even keener to spend time with both of them.

Bill Andrews, the brother of Mason Andrews and a Norfolk gynecologist who was also a subspecialist in infertility, had known Patrick Steptoe for some time. He offered to contact Patrick on our behalf to see if he could be persuaded to visit Norfolk to share knowledge and present a lecture to our faculty. Patrick agreed, and his visit was arranged for December of 1978.

It was only six months after Louise Brown's birth and at a time when our program was coming under initial attack in newspaper editorials and letters to the editor from people who objected to these new technologies. Although we were eager for Patrick's advice, we worried that the visit might be unwise if it inflamed our opponents and made our staff and supporters feel uncomfortable. In the end, we opted to go ahead, hoping that even die-hard objectors would never dare say that a healthy baby like Louise should never have been born. Besides Louise, there was now a second IVF baby from the British program: Alistair Macdonald who was born to a Scottish couple.

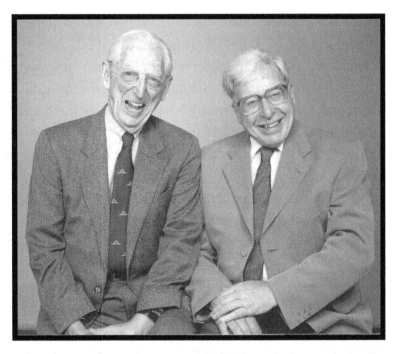

Howard Jones and Bob Edwards at a
reunion in Baltimore (2000).

That was the year when Patrick's contract as a National Health Service consultant had forced him into retirement because he reached the age of 65 in June. Bob attempted to pull all the stops, calling on pertinent contacts he knew in an effort to get the rule suspended, but the medical authorities were adamantly unmoved by appeals. The pair had no choice, short of opening a private clinic, to ensure that Patrick could continue providing clinical care to patients and carry on the practice of surgery.

Patrick and his wife, Sheena, decided to move closer to Cambridge and find premises near the university. After intense searching, Jean Purdy located a Jacobean mansion for sale some ten miles from Cambridge in a tiny village. When Bob and Patrick toured the stately home and its extensive gardens, they agreed it would make an ideal environment for their work away from prying eyes in the city, and surely a peaceful setting for patients. The location was Bourn Hall, which opened in 1980 as the first private clinic of its kind in the world.

Patrick's visit to Norfolk took place during his transition between Oldham and Bourn Hall. Perhaps our timing was lucky because it was almost a full year before his ultimate move to Cambridgeshire when he might have been too busy to accept our invitation. The visit and his lecture were great successes, and we learned much about their clinical techniques. Of greatest importance to me were his descriptions of laparoscopy, both its instrumentation and the timing for collection of oocytes, as well as his surprising use of nitrogen to inflate the abdomen. We adopted many of his recommendations, but by no means all. Only after he left did we realize that we had not asked him for their culture medium recipe, although we realized that was something that Bob and Jean were more familiar with.

Some years later, when I was talking to Ian Johnston (1930-2001), an Australian pioneer of IVF, he told me that he invited

Patrick to lecture in Melbourne. Evidently, the lecture was essentially the same as we had heard, but Ian's group too was disappointed that he skipped over lab details. It was an important omission because the viability of the gametes and embryos depended on the type of culture medium used during incubation. Ian had hoped to hear far more, especially after bringing Patrick and his wife in first class seats from London.

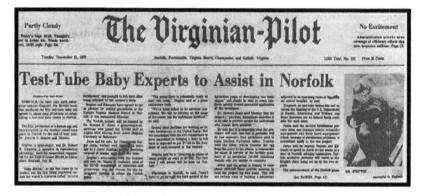

Patrick Steptoe gave a boost to our IVF program
when he visited Norfolk in November 1978,
shortly after the birth of Louise Brown.

On the day that Patrick stepped up to the podium in Norfolk for his open lecture at EVMS, he faced a full house and received a standing ovation afterwards. I remember he proposed nine steps for success in IVF.

1. The follicular phase of the menstrual cycle was ideally monitored by a combination of hormone measurements and ultrasound scanning.
2. The ovulatory surge of luteinizing hormone (LH) could be detected by urinary hormone assays.

3. Oocytes were best recovered by aspiration from the largest follicle(s) during laparoscopy.
4. In their program, oocytes were fertilized in a Petri dish.
5. The fertilized egg or "zygote" was checked at 2-, 4- and 8-cell stages.
6. Around the 8-cell stage the embryo(s) was transferred to the uterus for implantation.
7. The luteal phase should be monitored to check that menstruation had been suspended.
8. Pregnancy would be confirmed by a hormone test and detection of a fetal heart, and continued to be monitored by ultrasound.
9. Finally, the baby would be delivered.

Patrick ended his talk on an optimistic note affirming that IVF would take off in medical practice and spread around the world. That was prescient at a time when some critics were writing off the two IVF births to date as brief sensations. How satisfied he would be to know there are now about five million IVF babies in the world, and more every year.

We felt reassured that the visit had only positive effects and may have helped ease tensions in our region, and even countered local newspaper bias. Patrick and Sheena came to have dinner at our home one evening with a few of our colleagues. He described how Bourn Hall was being converted into a clinic by adapting the old rooms and adding new buildings for patient beds. Close by in the village, cottages had been bought for extra accommodation. He thought that IVF would remain an inpatient procedure and did not anticipate how rapidly it would change, making much of their investment redundant.

To our surprise, Patrick and his wife expressed interest in

our home and asked to look around. They thought the layout was exactly what they needed in England, which would include space for his grand piano (he was trained as a concert pianist), and asked us to mail them a copy of the house plan. A couple of years later when we were visiting Bourn Hall, Georgeanna and I saw their new home, but found it different and more attractive than our own.

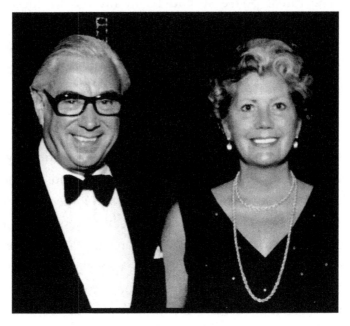

Patrick Steptoe and his wife Sheena.

As they were leaving, Patrick mentioned that he and Bob were presenting details of their program at a closed meeting of the Royal College of Obstetricians and Gynaecologists in London in January, 1979—only two months ahead. He said that there would be little that we had not already heard, but if we were interested, he would ask the college to send us an invitation. We would see two young Australian embryologists at the meeting who would soon become big names in the field—Alex Lopata and Alan Trounson. It was an invitation we could not refuse, although Georgeanna had to cancel. Jack Rary, who was then setting up our lab, came instead. He went ahead to enjoy a few days of sightseeing in London before the meeting at which we hoped to hear details about the mysterious culture medium.

My flight schedule was booked to arrive the day before the meeting so I would have a night to get over jetlag, but the winter weather did not cooperate. My first flight was from Norfolk to JFK in New York where I would change planes for an overnight passage to London where I was due to stay at Brown's Hotel which I knew from a previous trip. When the plane left Norfolk the morning of January 25, there was plenty of time in New York for the next leg of the journey. But it was raining and cloudy and, despite taking off on time, the visibility deteriorated, or at least that is how it appeared through the cabin window. It is normally only an hour to New York, but the captain announced that airport traffic control had instructed planes to circle until they were allowed to land. Thirty minutes later he announced that we had a low priority for landing and so we would have to fly to another airport to avoid running out of fuel! Philadelphia and other close major airports were not open to us and we continued to fly around. The passengers were quite uncomfortable by the time we eventually landed back in Norfolk, which we had left five hours before.

I called Georgeanna to pick me up at the airport, but while I waited the United Airlines ticket desk caught my eye. As the agent did not seem to have anything to do, I strolled across to ask if he had any suggestions as to how I might still get to London the next day. After a moment, he thought I might take the Concorde which was still flying the New York to London route. I booked the flight and, although very expensive, it would take only about three hours from JFK to my destination, so I could arrive around noon of the day before the meeting. In fact, I would land only slightly later than my original itinerary. I went home for a good rest and returned early the next morning for an uneventful journey.

However, my luggage failed to keep up with me. After checking in at Brown's Hotel in Mayfair, I asked the concierge for advice about hiring clothes. He could only think of a Bond Street tailor where I could be smartly outfitted for the day at the College. The next morning, I picked up a suit that would turn heads anywhere, even at the palace, and was back at the hotel by noon. My luggage had still not arrived. I asked Jack if I could borrow his electric razor but discovered he had overlooked the difference in European voltage: his razor would only fit American receptacles with 110 volts. Since Brown's is an upper crust hotel, I asked if it had a barber shop. There was one in the basement, so I hopped downstairs thinking it would be efficient to get a shave and a haircut at the same time. A professional shave was a new experience for me.

When I arrived, the only person in the shop was a bald man of some age who was sitting in a chair with his head in a newspaper. I assumed he was the barber because he wore a white jacket. When he stood up, he was short and his jacket dangled around his knees, reminding me of a senior physician making ward rounds.

He said, "You are very lucky today, sir. I'm generally booked in advance, but I just had a cancellation. Please take a seat."

He draped my shoulders with a cloth. "I will do the best I can," he said, doubtfully. "I guess your hairdresser in the States is a young, inexperienced man. If I had the chance to cut your hair two or three times I could make something of it." During the cut, he danced around my chair waving his scissors and comb, and backed off a few steps like a golfer lining up his putt. After combing my hair the last time, he picked up a bottle and started to sprinkle my head.

"This is a very special hair dressing," he said. "I make it with a secret formula. It will improve your hair. If you want to take some back to the States, I might be able to part with only a couple of bottles."

I bought them even though I was not sure I still possessed bags to pack for the homeward journey. I have forgotten the cost at the barber shop, except that it was considerable. It was good value as entertainment, even if the cut was indistinguishable from ones I have back home.

Back in my hotel room, I barely had time to dress for the meeting, which was scheduled to begin at 4:00 p.m. that afternoon at the Royal College. When I arrived, the long auditorium was already filling with men in dark suits whom I presumed were senior gynecologists and college fellows.

Patrick was the first speaker. He had spent most of his career in the north of England, far from the corridors of medical politics. That was not a career destination for most ambitious young doctors, yet he had suddenly become a doyen of reproductive medicine. He gave a comprehensive lecture in which he elaborated on the steps of IVF we already knew about. I listened closely to his description of how he retrieved oocytes from the ovary with a double-channel needle—one channel for aspirating the follicle and one for irrigating it afterwards to make sure it was evacuated.

I was particularly eager to hear Bob Edwards, who was billed to talk about laboratory procedures in the next lecture. He mentioned they used a standard culture medium (Eagles' Medium with Hanks' balanced salt solution), but did not specify whether it was used in the two cases that had pro-duced live births. His talk was otherwise heavy in scientific detail, and I recall him suggesting that estrogen and proges-terone secretion by cells from the follicle might predict the chances of pregnancy with the corresponding oocyte. His hunch was never confirmed, and identification of eggs with the highest pregnancy potential remains an unsolved problem to this day. Their two lectures were published in the college journal for a wider audience some eighteen months later.

Afterwards, there were doctors standing in the corridor asking why so few details about the culture medium had been presented. They too knew that fertilization and embryo growth depended on the recipe. We suspected that Patrick and Bob had to abide by some private agreement not to dis-close details of the technology in case it was patented, or per-haps because they were negotiating a contract to support their clinic.

Patrick and Sheena invited me, Jack Rary, and two other guests to dinner at an excellent restaurant in town. After a fine dinner and announcing that afternoon to the scientific world a revolutionary therapy for infertility that had evaded efforts down the ages, he stepped modestly into the rainy street wav-ing his arms. I can see him now asking a cab driver to take us back to the hotel. When I returned to my room, to my im-mense relief I saw my lost luggage lying on the floor beside the bed. What a day!

Although returning to Norfolk armed with new information, we continued to consult with anyone who had experience with *in vitro* fertilization. They were few and scattered across the globe. One of them was Pierre Soupart (1923-1981), a native of Belgium and professor of OB/GYN at Vanderbilt University.

We were unaware of his interests until he published articles in *Current Problems in Obstetrics and Gynecology* in 1979 in which he elegantly summarized everything that was then known of the technology. We quickly invited him to Norfolk for two or three days towards the end of that year.

Pierre became rather well-known for an episode arising from his application to the National Institutes of Health (NIH) for a research grant to investigate human fertilization and embryology. He submitted the grant in 1977, anticipating the emergence of clinical IVF by a full year. One of his aims was to test whether oocytes fertilized in an artificial medium were normal, which he planned to study by incubating oocytes and sperm together until he interrupted the process of fertilization for microscopic study. He hoped to confirm that fertilized eggs have a normal complement of 46 chromosomes.

The grant was approved by the NIH, but funding was held up by the Department of Health, Education, and Welfare (HEW) after it announced in January 1978 that an Ethical Advisory Board would be set up to review such work. The statement was unambiguous, so Pierre had to wait.

> *No application or proposal involving human in vitro fertilization may be funded by the Department or any component thereof until the application or proposal has been reviewed by the Ethical Advisory Board and the Board has rendered advice as to its acceptability from an ethical standpoint.*

The requirement seemed reasonable considering that researchers were entering controversial new territory but, intentionally or otherwise, the HEW created a significant roadblock since no Ethical Advisory Board had been instated, and the Secretary of HEW, Joseph Califano, delayed the appointment of a board for some unknown reason. After public pressure grew following the birth of Louise Brown, Secretary Califano eventually appointed one, and one of the first members happened to be the Reverend Richard McCormick, whom I later befriended. He later informed me about some of its actions. Their instructions were to draw up guidelines for evaluating grants and which restricted the study of human embryos in culture to a maximum of fourteen days. Grants for IVF research could be funded, but Soupart's application was still dangling, and in spite of being approved by both the NIH and the Advisory Board it was never funded. And he never pursued the project because he died in June 1981 at the early age of 58.

We were fortunate to have him as an advisor for a short while, although his recommendations did not alter our course. He told us he was aware of research on mice that indicated ambient light was harmful to fertilization, and that better results could be obtained with long wavelengths at the red end of the spectrum. Being cautious, Lucinda replaced fluorescent lights in the lab with incandescent light bulbs and fitted red filters on microscope lamps. But, as it was then more difficult to visualize eggs and embryos, we agreed to set aside this concern, which has not proven to be a problem in our program or elsewhere. Incandescent laboratory lighting still remains a standard practice.

Among our physicians, only Georgeanna was experienced with tissue culture techniques. When she was a medical student, she volunteered to be a technician in the Tissue Culture Laboratory at Hopkins which was then headed by George Gey (1899-1970). This was the laboratory where over a decade later he created the first line of immortal cancer cells from a cervical carcinoma in Henrietta Lacks. I was the surgeon who obtained the biopsies. The cells became famous as "HeLa cells;" they were first employed for developing a polio vaccine in the 1950s, and are still used today in medical research and drug development.

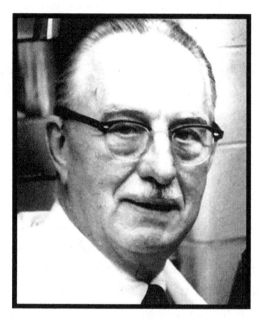

George Gey.

George's success may have been due to his invention of roller tubes, which he used to bathe cells in medium that was constantly but gently agitated. Georgeanna thought the same method, as opposed to static medium, might improve the development of embryos. Although there is little fluid in the fallopian tube, it is continually being stirred by tiny hairs (cilia) and by muscular contractions of the tubal wall, so that nutrients and oxygen is constantly refreshed around embryos. Lucinda began to study the problem by installing a shaker unit within an incubator chamber, but we abandoned the idea for lack of positive results. There is apparently no disadvantage to static medium, and Roger Gosden, an Edinburgh physiologist who trained in Cambridge under Bob Edwards, used a mathematical model to prove that human embryos can satisfy their nutritional needs by simple diffusion. Later on, Roger moved to join us at EVMS and subsequently married Lucinda. Lovely karma.

Two Australian groups were among Bob and Patrick's competitors. They had a great deal of experience after striving since 1973 to have the first IVF birth, though only with discouraging results, including an early miscarriage. I knew one of the leaders, Carl Wood, from an earlier visit to Melbourne, and after we started our program, I asked him if Anibal Acosta could spend a week in his clinic. After an arrangement was agreed, Anibal spent an additional week at another IVF program across town headed by Ian Johnston where the same embryologist was in charge, the gifted Alex Lopata. We returned the hospitality when Carl, and later Alex, visited us to share ideas and research news.

One of the innovations that Anibal brought home from his experience was to culture oocytes for at least four hours after recovery before insemination. This made perfect sense because it gave oocytes more time to complete maturation, but not so long that they risked becoming overripe. Another important difference in our laboratory protocols was to raise the pH of the culture medium from 7.2 to 7.4, the same as in blood.

Candace Reid was the first Australian IVF baby and third in the world. After her birth, there was a considerable gap until the next child arrived. Thus, there was very limited experience to go on when we started in 1980, and we were keenly aware that it had taken Edwards and Steptoe a decade of testing culture media and drugs before they had a protocol that actually worked.

Early on, some of their patients were treated with human menopausal gonadotropins, which consist of a mixture of follicle-stimulating hormone (FSH) and luteinizing hormone (LH) which are enriched in the urine after the menopause. Since these hormones stimulate follicle growth and estrogen secretion, it made sense to use them to stimulate patient's ovaries to harvest more oocytes and, hence, produce more embryos in hopes of improving the chances of pregnancy. Another advantage with gonadotropins was that, by overriding the endogenous hormones, the menstrual cycle was controlled and the time for retrieving mature oocytes was highly predictable.

The British group tested hormone treatment in about one hundred cases, but were never successful. They suspected that progesterone production was the problem. They switched back to untreated cycles, as in Australia, despite the obvious disadvantage that only one large follicle and therefore a single oocyte would be available. This made for problems when scheduling laparoscopy because of the need to be ready for action on a 24-7 basis.

Despite the obstacles, we adopted the same approach because of the greater experience of those groups. But Georgeanna doubted this was the best approach, as she had encountered the problem of timing ovulation in the natural cycle years earlier. She had extensive experience with the same gonadotropins when infertility was due to ovulation failure, and now pondered their value in IVF.

For her patients at Hopkins, she had to decide when they should schedule sexual intercourse or artificial insemination after hormone injections to ensure that sperm arrival in the upper reaches of the fallopian tube coincides with ovulation. If too early, the sperm would begin to degenerate before meeting the oocyte; if too late, the oocyte risked becoming overripe. She used the three methods then available for predicting when ovulation occurs: 1) basal body temperature, which rises promptly after ovulation from the effects of progesterone secretion, 2) the changed appearance and attachment of vaginal epithelial cells caused by high levels of estrogen, and 3) the appearance of mid-cycle cervical mucus when smeared across a glass slide, which appears fern-like (*spinnbarkeit*) under the influence of estrogen. Unfortunately, none of these methods predicted ovulation ahead of time, since they all came into full-bloom only after ovulation. We needed a more precise test.

We had a primitive ultrasound machine. It was serviceable for checking the progress of pregnancy by abdominal scanning, but almost useless for monitoring follicles which grow to the size of a large grape. Besides, visualization of ovarian follicles was hopeless in many of our early patients who had very serious pelvic disease with significant scarring.

However, by observing two "mock" menstrual cycles before the one in which oocytes were retrieved, we hoped to identify some characteristics for each patient that would be repeated in subsequent cycles, enabling us to know when to proceed. This idea was ultimately thwarted by human psychology because the treatment cycle proved less stable than prior ones, presumably because of the effects of stress on hormonal regulation.

We learned that British and Australian centers were using *Higonavis*, a Japanese hemagglutination test for LH, which was a predecessor of modern, super-sensitive enzyme-linked immunological tests (ELISAs). The advantage of this test was that the mid-cycle surge of LH occurs at a fixed interval *before* ovulation. Regrettably, three-hour urine samples had to be collected repeatedly for immediate analysis, and the test was fickle, expensive, and disruptive for patients and staff. Because of these issues, we decided to rely on the three biological "markers" I already mentioned, even though we knew they were all unsatisfactory.

We were also hampered in those days by gaps in knowledge of hormonal fluctuations of the menstrual cycle. We needed to determine the precise interval between the start of the LH surge and ovulation. After collecting samples from all 41 of our 1980 patients, we found that the surge lasts about 31 hours and ends soon after ovulation. Accordingly, we decided to aspirate follicles 28 hours after the LH surge began to be sure they had not already released their oocyte. That was a key piece of the puzzle, but many more pieces had to be tweaked before we were successful.

The efforts of 1980 were admittedly tentative and, at best, proved to be learning experiences. We retrieved only 19 oocytes from 41 women of which 13 were fertilized, but none of the embryos transferred established a clinical pregnancy.

Among our first cases that year, there was one in March that required laparoscopy at midnight, but it happened that snow had been falling heavily for the previous two days. Norfolk had already broken its all-time record for snowfall that winter, and now there was a white-out with 14 more inches expected, driven by gale force winds. Streets, schools, businesses, and the airport were closing, although the circus was still open and people and elephants trudged through snowy streets.

That weekend, Zev Rosenwaks, a young specialist from

New York, was visiting us with his wife and two children. He would later join our program, but on that Saturday we left my home together at 7:00 p.m., which allowed plenty of time to drive to our destination, only a couple of miles away. I packed a snow shovel in the trunk in case we got stuck, and we made a detour to pick up Anibal because he couldn't get his car out of the garage. The road conditions were so bad that we did not arrive at the hospital until 1:00 a.m. the next morning! By the time the remainder of the staff could be gathered for laparoscopy, it was about 3:30 a.m.

We were concerned that it was too late to collect the precious oocyte from the patient who had been monitored so carefully for weeks. She had probably ovulated already. When I had the laparoscope in position and could see the ovary, I confirmed that was the case. There was a trace of blood on the ovarian stigma where the oocyte had emerged through a rupture of the follicular wall. We had no idea of how far the oocyte had traveled after ovulation. I remember somebody suggesting that there was nothing to be lost by irrigating around the ovary with a balanced salt solution, and then inserting a larger needle supra-pubically in the faint hope that we could aspirate the injected fluid from the cul-de-sac. When this was done, Lucinda poured the fluid into a Petri dish to search under the microscope for an oocyte.

She announced that she had found it! I believe this was the first occasion, and maybe it is still the only time, that anyone has seen a freshly ovulated human oocyte. It was beautiful, seated inside a billowing cloud of sticky cells from the follicle, called cumulus granulosa cells. The oocyte was washed and transferred to the fertilization dish, but sadly never established a pregnancy. We did, however, learn something quite useful that night. Since the cell mass surrounding the oocyte was so large, it could not pass easily through the small needle we were advised to use without stripping off most of the cumulus cells adhering to the oocyte. Perhaps we were using too much suction pressure and too small a needle? Were we inadvertently damaging oocytes? Perhaps a small, but important change might enhance our patients' success with IVF. We decided there and then to use a larger needle and more gentle suction in the future.

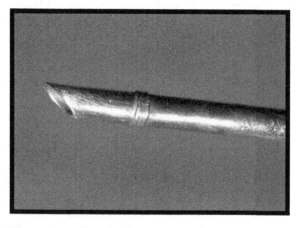

The "Blizzard needle" for harvesting oocytes from the ovary.

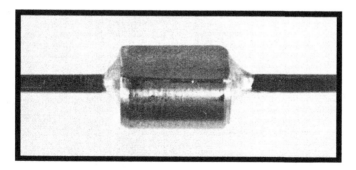

Turning the hub of the "Blizzard needle" to its flat side enabled the operator to know when its opening was inside the follicle.

I called an instrument maker I knew whom I had worked with at Hopkins. We designed what came to be known as the "Blizzard" needle, named in honor of the Norfolk storm that led to its construction. It was a larger 12 gauge needle with a cross-sectional area four times greater than one we had been using. We also designed a flattened rim about half an inch from the needle tip so that we could see how far inside the follicle the needle had penetrated. The new needle was much more efficient, and it was through trials and errors, like this example, that we groped our way forward.

6
BREAKTHROUGH

During the winter holiday break of 1980-1981, Georgeanna and I constantly reviewed our protocols and discussed them with other team members. There was still no breakthrough, and we struggled to decide which modifications might increase our chances of a pregnancy. After all this brainstorming, we made only two major changes: one was in the clinic and the other in the laboratory.

Despite Bob Edwards' warning not to use gonadotropins to stimulate the ovaries, Georgeanna insisted that we give it a try, even if it was going to complicate the routine for patients. A hormone preparation, called *Pergonal*, was available commercially, and she had used it to promote ovulation in women with infrequent cycles and in others who had stopped ovulating completely. There seemed no reason why it should not work in our patients who were menstruating normally, but the trick might be to administer a smaller dose than Bob had used. A dose of only one or two ampules a day for 3-4 days had enabled most of Georgeanna's patients to ovulate at Hopkins.

We began giving two ampules a day from about the fourth day of the menstrual cycle, continuing until the sixth or seventh day. Afterwards, we allowed the follicles to "coast" during the interval after injections until oocytes were retrieved. Follicle growth was monitored by ultrasound scanning. We were aiming to grow a single follicle to full size but, in fact, we often harvested from two, three, or even four follicles, and most of them contained a mature oocyte.

At 8:00 a.m. each day, the women had their blood drawn for measuring estrogen levels. Estrogen is mainly produced by the dominant follicle(s) and thus serves as an indicator of how far it has developed. Ultrasound played a role in monitoring treatment cycles, but it was not a central role until transvaginal scanning became available a few years later. Our older ultrasound transducer could only be used externally for visualizing the general appearance of ovaries, and didn't give us precise measurements needed for individual follicle diameter. Since ovaries are more visible with a full bladder, the patients would return to the waiting room after their blood was drawn to pour drinks from pitchers of water or lemonade. They filled their bladders until they were uncomfortable. When they were almost bursting, they called the nurse to take them for scanning. It sometimes happened, of course, that two people felt ready at the same moment, so one had to hop around until we could get her to the examination room.

We held daily meetings at 1:00 p.m. to review the morning blood and ultrasound tests, and determine the dose of *Pergonal* for each patient. As the team endocrinologist, Georgeanna organized these sessions, which she called "values." Every patient was discussed in turn to make the best decision for them, a routine which also served as an important learning experience for all of us. Patients returned to the clinic at 4:00 p.m. for hormone injections.

In her long experience with *Pergonal*, Georgeanna knew

that it was a very effective way of stimulating follicles to grow, but they often failed to ovulate. We encountered the same failure of ovulation in IVF patients on *Pergonal*, even in those who were ovulating normally before treatment. In the menstrual cycle, the leading follicle produces most of the estrogen which, when it reaches a certain threshold level, triggers a surge of luteinizing hormone (LH) from the pituitary gland. LH causes the final maturation of the oocyte and its ovulation. We therefore decided that after *Pergonal* had done its job we would give patients a second hormone—human chorionic gonadotropin (hCG). Pure LH was rare and expensive, but hCG was a biochemical mimic and readily available. It succeeded fabulously well.

This was a great blessing because it enabled us to precisely schedule the time of oocyte retrieval, and also helped to support the corpus luteum that forms from the collapsed follicle and produces progesterone to prepare the uterus for implantation of the embryo. Our research had already revealed the time from the onset of the LH surge to ovulation in the natural cycle, and we presumed it would be similar after administering hCG. We calculated that laparoscopy should be carried out 36 hours after hCG was injected, which gave us a couple of hours leeway before ovulation was expected. Hence, if a patient was injected on Monday night at 7:30 p.m., she would be scheduled for laparoscopic oocyte retrieval early on Wednesday morning. If we had, say, five patients ready at the same time, the Monday night injections would be given at hourly intervals.

We expected that most oocytes would be completely mature when they were retrieved (i.e., at metaphase II of maturation), but had taken the precaution advised by our Australian colleagues to culture them for a few hours before exposing them to sperm. This is because eggs are more likely to become abnormal or remain unfertilized if still immature when they are incubated with sperm. But it was difficult to verify oocyte maturity under the microscope since the dense cumulus cells surrounding the oocyte obscured the polar body and the anucleate cytoplasm that could confirm a mature status.

Being on call to give hormone injections around midnight was inconvenient for everyone involved, so we handily arranged with one of the nursing stations at the hospital to administer them at the assigned times. For patients, this meant they had to go to the hospital at night, but it had the advantage of familiarizing them with the place where they would soon undergo laparoscopic egg retrieval.

When patients were making daily treks to our offices, they had the opportunity of getting to know one other in the waiting room between sessions with clinical staff. It was often quite a collegial atmosphere as they exchanged their own stories and experiences. There was a coffee break at 10:00 a.m. when introductions were made and patients were given an opportunity to ask questions of the staff. I was surprised that so many questions revolved around reproductive physiology since a good many of our patients were quite well-educated. I understood then that our educational system was letting people down if so many reach adulthood, even with college degrees, without having the faintest notion of how eggs are formed, where fertilization occurs, and changes in the body during early pregnancy. Surely, such fundamental facts that underlie the survival of our species should not be confined to a physiology classroom.

By the end of 1981, treatment of twenty-four patients using the newly-refined stimulation protocols had progressed to the stage at which we could retrieve oocytes by laparoscopy.

Apart from one cycle in which a burr on the needle tip affected aspiration and another in which all the oocytes were immature, in every case we were able to generate fertilized eggs.

Strides were being made in the laboratory. There was a realization that extraordinary cleanliness and sterility were essential for cell culture and, in hindsight, this was an early step towards the controlled laboratory environment we take for granted today. Lucinda purged the lab of anything superfluous, and clutter was banned. A strict routine of hand-washing before entering the lab was established. Scrubs, masks, head coverings, and gloves were mandated at all times. She was equally obsessive in making culture medium by using the purest chemicals available and distilling water four times before use. Although gametes and embryos are never exposed to light in their natural environment, we had put this anxiety to test, although only allowing low levels of illumination in the laboratory. With more confidence, we even began taking photographs in culture, and to this day patients are given pictures of their embryos that we hope will become their baby's first portrait. One of the first embryos photographed became our first IVF baby. Over the years, Lucinda published four highly-illustrated atlases of gamete and embryo development, and developed techniques for assessing oocyte maturation, embryo grading, and sperm isolation.

During that year, we also devoted a great deal of effort to developing a computer database for clinical and research purposes. One must recall that these were very early days for using a technology that is so widely familiar today. We were incredibly fortunate to have a smart and enthusiastic OB/GYN resident at the hospital by the name of Charles Wilkes. He knew more about computers and computer programming than anyone else with whom we were acquainted at the time.

I had initially gotten to know Charlie after he interviewed for our residency program in 1979. Picking up on the fact that he possessed a passion for computer programming, he seemed a natural fit to help our new program grow in an organized manner. He initially demonstrated to me a database program written in BASIC, which was impressive enough to spur us into purchasing our first computer early in 1981. That computer was an Apple II with a whopping 8K memory, but essentially the first commercially available personal computer. Later, writing in a computer language called APL and working with an IBM XT, he managed to improve and expand an extensive database that allowed us to assess and refine the efficacy of our clinical protocols, track patient responses and outcomes, and fine tune newly-introduced laboratory methods. He also worked with Lucinda to update and improve software for collecting data. Our computers were regularly upgraded, and always with Charlie's recommendations and valued assistance. When the day eventually arrived for mandatory submission of clinic-specific data to an external oversight agency, our program was ahead of the pack in computer readiness.

Judith Carr, a 27-year-old from Massachusetts, was our thirteenth patient and sixth transfer after introducing all these changes. She came with a history of three ectopic pregnancies after an earlier bout of acute appendicitis. At the first ectopic pregnancy, her tube and the ovary on the same side were removed. At the second, the surgeon managed to preserve the remaining tube after removing the conceptus implanted inside it, hoping that it could function normally. However, a third ectopic pregnancy occurred in that tube at which time it was removed. She, therefore, had no possibility whatsoever of becoming pregnant without medical assistance, which seemed beyond reach.

On the day that her specialist told her the bad news, there was a newspaper article in a local paper reporting that doctors in Norfolk were trying to fertilize eggs *in vitro* for bypassing the need for fallopian tubes when they were blocked or absent. This specialist had been stationed as a gynecologist at one time at the Portsmouth Naval Hospital, across the Elizabeth River from Norfolk, so the article meant more to him than it might otherwise. He handed her the article with advice to think about it. Judy Carr and her husband, Roger, had read about the birth of Louise Brown in England, but did not connect that news with her own circumstances. In her own words: "[IVF] was not even a blip on my radar screen." She applied to our program and was accepted because she matched all our criteria, being healthy, under 35 years old, and lacking fallopian tubes. The procedure she was about to undertake was at that time illegal in the state of Massachusetts where they lived.

Her treatment began in early May, two or three days before we were due to fly to Europe. Georgeanna was invited speak at a French society for OB/GYN specialists about the luteal phase defect. We decided to accept an oft-repeated invitation to visit Bourn Hall *en route* to Paris. Since we could not get a reservation in Bourn village, we stayed at the Old Bridge Hotel in Huntingdon, some miles away in Cambridgeshire.

The day was spent with Patrick in the operating theater, which is what the O.R. is called in the UK, and a good part of the next day we were in the lab with Bob. Afterwards, Patrick and Sheena took us out to a princely meal at a restaurant in the City of Cambridge, so we returned to our hotel room rather late, around 11:00 p.m. As that corresponded to 6:00 p.m. Eastern Standard Time, I called Norfolk to speak to Jairo

Garcia for news of our patients. I told him I was mystified why none of them had become pregnant, because there was nothing that the Brits were doing that was substantially different to us, as far as I could see. His reply startled me.

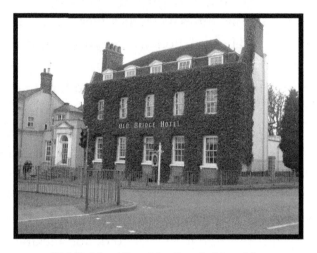

Old Bridge Hotel in Cambridgeshire.

"I think we have one."

He told me that Judy Carr had missed her period and was continuing in the luteal phase because her basal temperature was still elevated. I had transferred an embryo to her just before leaving for Europe. She was only two days overdue for her period, so this was a very tentative sign, and just a bit too early for a pregnancy test in those days. Nevertheless, when Georgeanna and I flew out of Heathrow the next morning, we were cautiously optimistic.

On arrival around noon at the Sofitel Bourbon Hotel in Paris, there was a note waiting for us at the reception desk asking for a call back to our office. When I got through to the secretary, she recognized my voice. She said that, although she was instructed not to tell, she could not hide the news that

Judy's blood test was positive. We were so elated that we decided to celebrate at a wonderful little Parisian restaurant with the best meal in the house. The meal cost both of us the equivalent of only about $50 in 1980, but today I guess it would be nearer to $200.

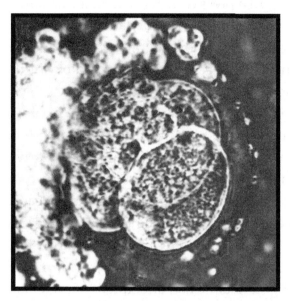

The early cleavage-stage embryo that was transferred to Judy Carr which resulted in the birth of Elizabeth.

At the conference, we came across an old friend, Jean Cohen, in whom we confided news of our first IVF pregnancy. He told us this was a great coincidence because a French program had recently announced at a press conference that they had a positive pregnancy test. The patient had then been besieged by reporters and shortly afterwards suffered a miscarriage. It could never be proved to have been caused by the hullabaloo, but Jean advised us in the best interests of our patient to keep the news, or at least her identity, private for as long as possible.

On our return to Norfolk, we were met by Jairo and Mason and Sabine Andrews, but instead of going straight home we sat down with our bags at the airport to catch up with the news. That day happened to be Mother's Day, and they had a special Mother's Day card for us. After some discussion, we decided to hold a press conference to make an announcement, but would conceal Judy's identity and address.

A press conference the following Monday filled a small room at the medical school. After my statement that we had a pregnancy, the reporters leaned over to scribble rapidly on their notepads for they knew that the first IVF baby in America was big news and wanted to catch every crumb of information. But would they respect our appeals for privacy and, if not, would they be able to find Judy? I mentioned that a woman in Paris who conceived after IVF had a miscarriage which might have been caused by the publicity. I think my message got through because the press never identified her, although I had my doubts about press integrity confirmed when a reporter admitted that he had attempted to locate her. We owed her security to the discretion of our staff and the fact of her living several hundred miles north of Norfolk.

As the pregnancy progressed without complications, we talked with her over the phone and amongst ourselves in closed sessions to decide where she should deliver her baby. A decision dangled for a long time, although the general hope in our group was it would be in Norfolk.

It so happened that June 1981 was the fiftieth anniversary of my graduation from Amherst College, and I wanted to attend the reunion. As it was not a long drive from Amherst to Westminster, Massachusetts, where the Carrs lived, I took the opportunity to visit them to discuss arrangements for the delivery. We unanimously agreed on Norfolk. Meanwhile, she would commute between Westminster and our clinic for prenatal checkups, with Mason Andrews as her obstetrician. The plan went without a hitch. I would drive Judy from the airport to his office, and she would stay overnight at a hotel under an assumed name. No one outside our tight circle ever knew.

In August, I had a telephone call from Gordon Stevens who was a business manager for Peter Williams at an independent British broadcasting firm. Peter was a well-known producer of TV documentaries in which he appeared as an interviewer and narrator. He knew about our *in vitro* program from Bob Edwards, who had supplied our names and addresses when he was taping a story at Bourn Hall Clinic. Peter wanted to come to Norfolk to discuss the possibility of recording our operation, but since Georgeanna and I were returning to England in a couple of weeks, I suggested we meet near London.

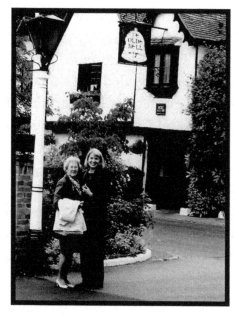

Georgeanna Jones and Lucinda Veeck at
Ye Olde Bell in the early 1990s.

The meeting took place at Ye Olde Bell in Hurley, Berkshire, reputed to be the oldest working inn in the country (Twelfth Century). We had stayed there several years earlier because it was convenient for early morning flights from Heathrow Airport. We discussed the proposition over dinner with Peter and Gordon, and agreed to go ahead. Since they only knew we had an IVF program, they were very excited to hear that we now had a pregnancy and were even more eager to press ahead. They departed from the hotel early the next morning before we were down for a traditional English breakfast, and when we appeared at the desk to check-out, we found they had paid our bill. That generosity seemed a tangible confirmation of sincere interest in our story.

Gordon came to Norfolk in October to meet officials at the hospital and medical school, and to make arrangements for the film crew. In November, a group of six photographers, an editor, and sound recorder arrived to tape one of Judy's prenatal visits. They returned on Monday, December 28 of 1981 for her delivery by Cesarean-section.

The O.R. was a very crowded place that day. Besides our staff, there was an expectant father and the film crew who had perched cameras and lights at strategic places around the room. Mason Andrews was in charge, assisted by two residents, Charlie Wilkes (our computer guru) and Clarke Bundren. Quincy Asque was one of the pair of anesthesiologists who had offered to help if a need arose, as it did now. Fred Wirth, a pediatrician, was in attendance, and Doris Gentilini was the standby or "circulating" nurse. All the other physicians and embryologists in our team were present including, of course, Georgeanna and myself.

We hoped that Judy would have a normal vaginal delivery, but ultrasound scans revealed the head of the baby was at the lower limit of normal in its biparietal diameter (a measure of skull size). At that time, it was one of the few non-invasive tests available for predicting intrauterine viability. The small size worried us and led to our decision to go for a C-section.

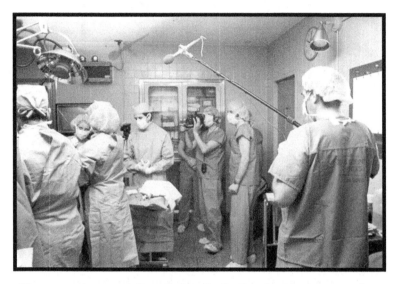

The operating room just before Judy Carr's Cesarean section.

To say I was uneasy is an understatement of how I really felt. The day before, I drafted a fallback press release stating the patient was doing well, but her baby was found to be abnormal and I appealed that her privacy be respected. I added we had two more patients with ongoing pregnancies whom we hoped would be normal in every way. In the event, my anxieties were needless because Baby Elizabeth was not only beautiful, but perfectly normal. Georgeanna never shared my misgivings; she predicted a good outcome because both the mother and father possessed small frames.

Thankfully, there were only a few reporters around that day. After the delivery, we made a simple announcement that the baby was born without complications and was healthy. A formal press conference was announced for the same morning at 11:00 a.m.

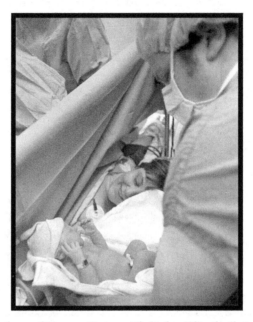

Judy and Roger Carr with Baby Elizabeth two minutes old and still inside the operating room.

Georgeanna and I went home to prepare for it, but she needed to stop by a beauty parlor because her hair was a "mess." We did not get home until about 10:00 a.m., and no sooner had we gotten inside when the telephone rang. It was Ian Craft, a long-time friend and gynecologist in London. Our news had raced across the ocean to be broadcasted by the time Americans were just waking up to it. I was absolutely flabbergasted at the speed of modern communications which we so take for granted today.

The press conference was arranged in the hospital by

Vernon Jones, the part time public relations officer who had drafted a statement for me. It read:

> *It's a girl! At 7:43 a.m. this morning, Elizabeth Jordan Carr, the daughter of Mr. and Mrs. Roger Carr of Westminster, Massachusetts, was delivered successfully by a Cesarean section by Dr. Mason Andrews. Dr. Frederick Wirth, the pediatrician, says Elizabeth is quite normal.*

Standing at the front of the room with our staff behind me, I explained that because Judy had been delivered by C-section, she could not be present at the conference that day. If all went well she would attend another press meeting.

On that second occasion, Roger and Judy with Baby Elizabeth were escorted into the room to rapturous applause and tears of joy in which even some of the press shared. Judy made a statement of appreciation to everyone involved, but declined to answer questions at that time as she was tired and feeling overwhelmed. In a private moment, Roger admitted: "Such a feeling of relief and joy that the journey is over and we have finally been blessed." Georgeanna and I agreed along with so many others that we were indeed fortunate to have the Carrs as our first parents, as they were both so gracious and appealing in the midst of intense public scrutiny.

Though questions to Judy would be put off until another day, the press was not barred from firing them at the medical team behind the front table. They wanted to hear all the fine details about how the pregnancy and delivery had progressed. We were able to reply affirmatively in every instance, although we admitted an earlier concern about the size of the baby, and mentioned the draft statement we never had to use. Dr. Wirth confirmed the baby was making excellent progress, and Elizabeth remained alert and never cried or whimpered at the conference. She absolutely stole the show.

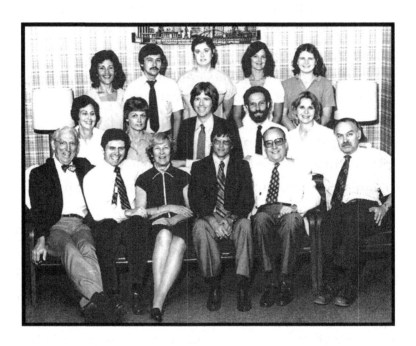

The medical team responsible for the first birth after IVF (names left to right). 1st row: Howard Jones, Jairo Garcia, Georgeanna Jones, Edward Wortham, Anibal Acosta, George Wright. 2nd row: Doris Gentilini, Nancy Garcia, Clark Bundren, Bruce Sandow, Lucinda Veeck. 3rd row: Margaret Whitfield, Charlie Wilkes, unknown, Linda Lynch, Jeannine Witmeyer. A most important member is missing–Dr. Mason Andrews, who performed the Cesarean section on Judy Carr.

The event was covered widely by local and national news media, with over a hundred editorials, and Peter Williams' documentary, *A Daughter for Judy*, was aired on PBS as a NOVA Special on January 27, 1982. The hospital collected press clippings for our records, all of which were very favorable except for one in a Norfolk newspaper. This editorial and letters to the editor that followed caused us a lot of grief and continued for several months.

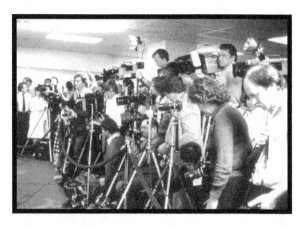

Press conference in Norfolk (December 31, 1981).

The first opportunity to present our breakthrough at a scientific meeting was in March 1982 at the American Fertility Society in Las Vegas. After describing the history of our program and the Carr conception and delivery, I pointed out that we still had great difficulty deciding whether an embryo had pregnancy potential based on morphological appearance. This was, and continues to be, a problem when there are multiple embryos available from which to choose one or two for transfer.

During cleavage divisions, embryonic blastomeres often become distorted, and it is difficult to distinguish normal from abnormal embryos based on a single microscopic evaluation. To illustrate the point, I showed a slide of an embryo I had transferred at an early stage. I invited anyone in the audience to predict if this one was normal or abnormal, and promptly recognized the man who stood up to take the challenge. The

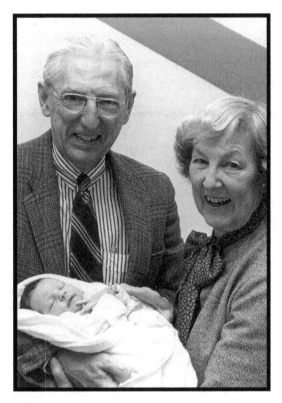

Howard and Georgeanna Jones admire
their first "IVF granddaughter."

gentleman was a distinguished professor of physiology who had made the first time-lapse films of ovulation in animals and was a former president of the society. He was certain that the embryo would never grow to be a viable fetus. When I revealed that it was the embryo that had led to the birth of Elizabeth Carr, he became very disturbed and did not speak to me again for several years. He was a known opponent of clinical IVF in those days .

Our second successful IVF pregnancy took a peculiar turn. The patient sought help in Norfolk after hearing about our program, but also in part to avoid gossip in her home town.

More than thirty years ago, the inability to have children was still an embarrassing subject, and couples were uncomfortable admitting they had a problem.

As this patient's pregnancy approached full term, she elected to deliver her baby at a large medical center close to her home. This was fine with me, but I urged her to be delivered by Cesarean section because she had had a bilateral salpingectomy with wedge resections where the fallopian tubes are attached to the uterus. I was concerned that her uterus might rupture at one or both of the original incisions during birth. She would then probably lose her uterus, perhaps the baby too, and never again carry a pregnancy.

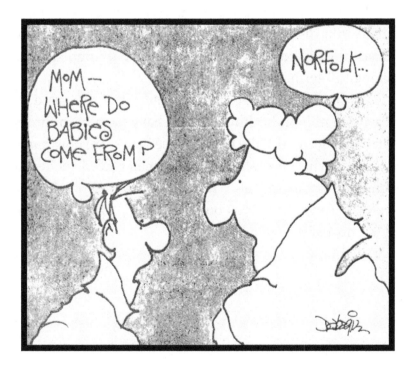

Sitting in my office one day, I received a phone call from an excellent obstetrician whom I knew who had just delivered that patient by C-section. While suturing the uterine wound, he was amazed that he could not find any tubes, but he knew that she had been treated in Norfolk. He made the call from the O.R. while the patient was still lying on the table with her abdomen open.

"What is going on?" he asked. "What should I do?"

I told him not to worry but simply close the abdomen. He had not heard about IVF, but soon those three letters would be on the lips of most practitioners and patients alike.

Progress was accelerating. Nineteen treatment cycles in 1981 had established five pregnancies, all of which were carried to term. Success rates were improved by transferring more than one embryo, which only became possible after we started using ovarian stimulation. Transferring one embryo resulted in a disappointing 13% delivery rate, but with two embryos it climbed to 31%, and with three it jumped to 50% reaching full-term.

Now, more than three decades later, it is estimated that at least five million healthy children have been born through IVF technologies. And the first of those babies are now parents themselves who generally have no greater need for fertility treatment than anyone else. Judy and Roger Carr are grandparents to Trevor who was born August 5, 2010 to Elizabeth and her husband, David Comeau.

7

A SUIT FOR LIBEL

It was rather poignant that the main opposition to our IVF program was our own local newspaper, the *Virginian Pilot,* and even more ironic that when Elizabeth Carr grew up, she served for six months as an intern journalist for that paper. The letters column frequently published comments affirming its policy of opposition to our program. Charles Dean was one of the regular correspondents around the time Elizabeth was born, and he became highly visible around the campus wearing a sandwich board, which declared, "See Me for the Truth." He handed out pamphlets to pedestrians, hoping to recruit any who might be sympathetic to his views.

We felt somewhat reassured when the paper's editor pointed out that IVF babies had already been born in England and Australia, although the numbers were stated inaccurately. The editor predicted that the practice would probably expand, with which we agreed. The rest of the article outlined the rudiments of reproductive physiology and mentioned that, because the process is inefficient, only about one in five fertilized eggs normally implants. To that extent, we had some common ground with the newspaper, which seemed to be adopting a neutral stance in that it neither supported nor condemned IVF.

But the very next day, the editorial section was in quite a different tone. It stated that a halfway house existed near the hospital for housing children suffering from various defects and where they received treatment. It pointedly accused that "those doctors involved in the IVF program at the hospital" would never accommodate a child at the halfway house because they had decided that patients suspected during pregnancy of having an abnormal baby would come under pressure to have an abortion. We were horrified to read this scurrilous story since it was totally false. We were also puzzled why the editorial tone had reversed from the previous day.

A couple of days later, I received a call from Robert Nusbaum, a local attorney I knew only slightly, but who was a longtime friend of Mason Andrews. He wanted to come to my office on campus to discuss the newspaper article. Bob was very excited about Elizabeth's birth and expressed deep interest in our work, but the hostile editorial distressed him. He said it was unlikely that there would be a change of policy at the newspaper unless some positive action was taken. And he added that the second editorial, published on December 31, had all the hallmarks of libel.

Bob explained that when the reputation of people is maligned in print with the knowledge that it is inaccurate, the court will presume that statements are libelous. He had reason to believe from an employee at the paper that the editor had been warned before publication that the story about patients with abnormal babies was inaccurate. His source had urged the author to check his facts before going to print, but for some reason that precaution was overlooked and the draft moved forward unchanged.

The only possibility open for stopping further harassment, as far as Bob could see, was to sue the newspaper. Mason, Anibal, Jairo, Georgeanna, and I gathered to discuss all the implications of bringing a suit against an influential local paper. None of us had experience of court proceedings but, confident in Bob's counsel, we decided unanimously to proceed.

The reference to "those doctors" in the article implied the five physicians, but he advised us against banding together to bring the suit. He thought it was better if only one of us was involved in the case, and if things went well in the preliminary stages the other four could join afterwards.

He recommended we choose the person who would seem to the court to be the least belligerent. "Who should that person be?" he asked. It was hard to ask Georgeanna to take on that role, but she was the obvious choice.

It was not necessary to name a sum for the compensation sought at the preliminary filing of our suit, because this would be decided when, or if, we reached the point of going to trial. The award would be scaled according to the defendant's assets, which would be disclosed at that time. Furthermore, if we had to propose a nominal amount for compensation it could still be changed later. Thus, on December 9, 1982, Georgeanna filed a suit as a plaintiff against the *Virginian Pilot* for $5,500,000.

Over the next three to four months while the wheels were turning, we were learning the ins and outs of the legal system. There were technical terms, like *discovery* and *depositions*, that many of us had never heard of before, but they became more familiar from meetings with Bob and lawyers from the other side held in the presence of a court recorder. All members of the team with relevant knowledge were asked to give evidence under oath, and most of us were called to attend two meetings.

I cannot recall feeling uncomfortable on any occasion, and I thought the experience was rather interesting. The lawyers wanted to know the nuts and bolts of how IVF was done, and were particularly anxious to find out if we ever had a discussion with our patients about pregnancy termination because that was, of course, the crux of what we were being accused of. We could easily answer that question because there never had been such a discussion, and that was that!

We were also asked about the policy of the British group, which made our attorney, Bob Nusbaum, uneasy. The defense wanted to know if it had required their patients to agree to undergo amniocentesis to determine if the fetus was normal and, if not, whether the pregnancy would have been terminated. Bob hesitated to allow us to answer, but eventually signaled for me to go ahead. I had the most extensive first-hand knowledge of Bourn Hall, and simply replied that, to my knowledge, there had been never such a discussion with any patient.

After the final meeting, the date was fixed for a hearing. Bob felt confident that our case was going smoothly, so he recommended the other four members of the team join the suit as co-plaintiffs alongside Georgeanna. As a group, we sued the newspaper for $27,500,000 .

Soon after the trial date was set, I received a call from Henry Clay Hofheimer, the businessman mentioned in an earlier chapter who was affectionately known as "Mr. Norfolk." He came to our home with Bob Payne, a leading surgeon in the city who was interested in civic affairs. Bob Nusbaum came too.

Henry Clay was worried that that the lawsuit was

beginning to divide the city, and many people were choosing sides for or against us. He hoped we might find a way to prevent the matter going to trial, and had a proposal. Would it be agreeable, he asked, if he and Dr. Payne approached Frank Batten, the newspaper owner, with the aim of settling the quarrel by arranging a meeting between Frank and Georgeanna?

Bob Nusbaum was confident that we would win at trial. We had already decided that in the event of any award, either from a suit or a settlement, all the money would be transferred to the EVMS Foundation to start a research fund. However, we eventually agreed that we should try to reach an amicable agreement with the newspaper by accepting Henry Clay's offer to act as a mediator.

After the meeting, Georgeanna explained what happened in the Hofheimer office. She had begun by apologizing to Mr. Batten for causing him so much difficulty since he had not personally authored the offending editorial. If the row had occurred with the *Baltimore Sun*, she said that we would have gone directly to the owner, whom we knew, thus avoiding the threat of court proceedings. Mr. Batten made a courteous reply in return. He explained that, on the contrary, it was he who needed to apologize. In fact, he thought that IVF should proceed in Norfolk and the paper was prepared to make a settlement.

In due course, a two-part settlement was agreed upon. First, there was the financial side, which was never to be disclosed and, second, the newspaper would print a retraction and apologize for the earlier editorial. There were several drafts before Bob received what he thought matched the situation, and recommended that we accept the terms.

When the settlement money was received by the plaintiffs, we turned it over to the medical school as planned, and it supported our research for several years. I have often said that if one is looking for research funds it is easier to win a suit for libel than to write grant applications to the National Institutes of Health, which generally have slim chances of success.

Bob predicted, however, that opposition to our program would continue through other channels, which turned out to be correct. But opposition from the *Virginian Pilot* ceased. Mr. Batten replaced Terry Eastland, the author of the defamatory editorial, and made other managerial changes at the paper which subsequently became a supporter of our efforts and the practice of IVF more generally.

8

IN THE VATICAN CITY

After several healthy IVF babies were conceived in our program, the first being Elizabeth Carr, we were confident of mastering the technology. As news spread, we received many requests from people seeking training at all levels, and invitations to speak at meetings around the world. One of those invitations was received from Professor Silvio Bettocchi in Bari, Italy, in 1983. Silvio wanted Georgeanna and me to attend a national meeting along with other professors of obstetrics and gynecology who wanted to introduce IVF to Italy. We noticed the conference guest list included Monsignor Carlo Caffarra (1938-), although his significance was not apparent until sometime later.

Monsignor Caffarra worked in the Vatican where he was appointed by the Pope as President of the John Paul II Institute for Studies on Marriage and Family. The conference organizers in Bari probably hoped that if they could secure his approval at the outset of their endeavors, it would be very beneficial for future growth of IVF in the country. If that was their calculation, it badly misfired because he was known, even within his church, as an arch-conservative and fierce critic of artificial birth control methods. We did, however, have interesting discussions with the Monsignor during the conference and in private when we had meals together.

He protested against the practice of IVF because he thought it would promote abortion, which was an objection we had heard before at the Halloween Day hearing in Norfolk. This was only his general concern. What really troubled him was that conception *in vitro* was conducted outside the bonds of conjugal love. We did not realize the gravity of his criticism at the time because we were focused on scientific and medical issues, and were making arrangements at the conference for hosting trainees from Italy. When we returned to the country the following year, we understood we had a problem.

Early in 1984, Georgeanna and I received identical letters postmarked Rio de Janeiro with the letterhead of the Pontifical Academy of Sciences; they were signed by the academy's president, Carlos Chagas Filho (1910-2000). He wrote that in the fall of the same year, the academy planned to host a meeting in the Vatican Gardens to discuss IVF. He expressed a hope that we would accept an invitation if one were to be sent by the Vatican.

As I was receiving all sorts of correspondence during those years, I had some doubts about the genuineness of the letter, especially since I had never heard of the Pontifical Academy. Neither of us responded to the letters immediately because I was wary in case someone was trying to fool us. But the more I thought about them, the more I guessed they were legitimate. The name Carlos Chagas was not unfamiliar to us as physicians because Chagas Disease was named eponymously for the famous Rio microbiologist who had discovered it. I guessed there was a connection with the author of the letter, as indeed there was. He was Chagas' son, and he had followed his father into the medical sciences to become a distinguished Brazilian biophysicist. In the days before the Internet was at our fingertips, it took longer to check information, so I chose the quickest route for verifying the authenticity of the letters by inviting to dinner the chaplain at the DePaul Hospital in Norfolk.

When I showed him the letters, he became very excited and confirmed they truly were from the Pontifical Academy. He explained that it had been founded by the church as a successor to the 1603 Accademia dei Lincei to promote a better understanding of science and avoid repeating the fiasco of suppressing Galileo's championing of theories about the universe. He told me that groups of experts are assembled in the Vatican from time to time to inform moral theologians about progress in science and technology before they in turn advise the Holy See. I wondered if we were on the invitation list because Monsignor Caffarra remembered us from the meeting in Bari the year before. We no longer hesitated to send replies to Professor Chagas, and a formal invitation arrived soon afterwards. The meeting would be held in the Casina Pius IV of the Vatican Gardens in October.

The Casina is a beautiful summer house of white marble which Pope Pius IV created to escape the heat of his quarters three hundred yards away. It was later converted to the headquarters of the Pontifical Academy.

Georgeanna and I stayed at the Michelangelo Hotel inside the Vatican compound where we dined in the large refectory. As a man without a clerical collar and with a woman, I felt completely out of place, and as we were escorted to our table, the buzz of conversation in the room hushed until we sat down. We often overheard people at other tables referring to "J. P.," which puzzled us at first. After a few times, we realized this was their nickname for John Paul II, although we courteously referred to him by the title, *His Holiness*.

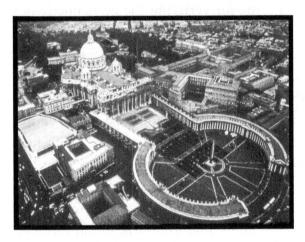

The Pontifical Academy of Sciences met in the building to the right of the dome of St. Peters at The Vatican.

On the first morning, we were met by a driver who took us halfway around the outskirts of the Vatican wall to enter a gate to the Casina Pius IV. The executive director, Monsignor Enrico di Rovasenda, was there to welcome us. The other eight men attending were distinguished doctors, scientists, or moral theologians, and most of them were polyglots. There was only one other gynecologist beside ourselves—René Frydman from Paris.

Monsignor di Rovasenda explained official protocol for our stay. He said we would be referred to as, "Your Excellencies," although, in fact, no one ever used the term in our presence. In the event of an ecclesiastical procession, we would march with other members of the academy behind the cardinals and in front of the bishops. That we were given such a privilege impressed me, and I mischievously imagined parading ahead of Bishop William Sullivan of the Archdiocese of Richmond, who had expressed such great disappointment in our work.

The location within the Vatican Gardens was fabulous. We were able to relax during coffee breaks under a marble porch adjacent to the Sistine Chapel which, for all its amazing art inside, looked rather drab outside and was closed for major restoration work at that time. Monsignor Caffarra offered to take us on a private tour of the chapel, but somehow during the busy program it never happened.

I expected meetings to open with prayers, but they never offered any, nor did they say grace before meals. We simply sat down to an abundance of excellent food and Italian red wine served by nuns who, we were told, had come with the Pope from Poland.

Professor Chagas informed us that the meeting would be recorded and, since Casina walls "don't have ears," we should openly express our personal views whether IVF was "licit" and harmonious with Catholic doctrine. We would have an opportunity to check the transcript for accuracy before it was published. He said our collective views would weigh heavily when the pontiff came to decide if IVF could be recommended for church members around the world.

The meeting was spread over three days. We were there to explain the medical background of IVF technology, and were limited to speaking in English. We lost the thread of conversation when members of the group shifted from English to one language and then another. On the second day, we were provided with a translator to sit between us and quietly render in our own tongue what was being said. He was so consummate a linguist that when people slipped back to English, he often switched to another language automatically.

Our translator turned out to be none other than Jerome Lejeune (1926-1994), the man who discovered the chromosomal basis for Down syndrome. He was a lifetime member of the academy and happened to be at the Vatican at the time. He is also the man quoted by Charles Dean in his ardent letter of protest which was widely circulated before we received approval to open our doors. Professor Lejeune was held in deep respect by everyone in attendance, and we heard that he took morning prayers with the Pope when he was in Rome.

On the third day, we sat in rapt attention when Professor Chagas asked the ordained members of the group whether IVF should be considered licit or illicit. That was a decisive moment in our proceedings. As he went around the table, the theologians said that if a parishioner came asking for the procedure they would say it was licit, but when he came to Monsignor Caffarra there was a dissenting voice. He declared IVF was illicit because it was "outside the bonds of conjugal love," as he had stated before. His argument was followed by a lively discussion to figure out exactly what he meant by that. His definition of conjugal love turned out to be sexual intercourse. When Chagas was unable to persuade Caffarra to change his position, he asked him if he could remain silent. Caffarra declined and warned he had the right ear of the Pope.

Our group had been promised a visit by His Holiness on the opening day, but it didn't happen. We were transferred to another location inside the Casina because our room was required for signing a treaty between Chile and Argentina over a border dispute in which the he had arbitrated. I was amazed to hear that Twentieth Century popes are still occupied with secular matters just as their predecessors were in centuries past. We never saw the Pope, although his greeting and blessing were relayed to us through Professor Chagas.

I wrote the above narrative from memory some years after our visit, but later found a summary that I composed soon after returning from the Vatican and had distributed to staff members. It contains some duplication of the story but, for the historical record, it is transcribed below in virtually unedited form.

The so-called 'working group' on 'Extracorporeal Fecundation' consisted of eleven individuals. In addition to the eleven invited people, Professor Carlos Chagas, President of the Pontifical Academy, was present and presided. Professor Chagas is a Brazilian and son of Carlos Chagas, who discovered the spirochete which causes Chagas disease and is very endemic in certain South American countries. Professor Chagas is perhaps seventy-six years old, and very keen. He had an extraordinary ability from time to time to halt the proceedings and summarize, and was able to focus on the important points, because during the discussion, there was a tendency for the various participants to stray from the subject. The meeting lasted for three days.

A word about the participants:

Professor Baumiller is the Jesuit priest who is responsible for the Genetics Division of the Department of Obstetrics and Gynecology at Georgetown University. He did his genetic training at Hopkins and runs the laboratory for Georgetown University.

Professor Adriano Bompiani was present only one day and he is chairman of the Department of Gynecology and Obstetrics at the Catholic University in Italy.

Mons. Prof. Carlos Caffarra is president of the Pontifical

John Paul II Institute for the Study of Matrimony and Family in the Vatican City. We met him in Bari.

Professor Luigi Carenza is chairman of the Department of Obstetrics and Gynecology at the University of Rome and is the chairman of the department who sent Giulietta to Norfolk (the same department in which Giovanni Sadurny works). He was present for only one session.

Professor René Frydman is well known to the members of the team, and he is the director of the in vitro program at the Hospital Beclere in France.

Professor Jerome Lejeune is the discoverer of the fact that Down syndrome was due to G-21 trisomy. He is a well-known, extremely conservative Catholic geneticist who is opposed to aborting G-21 trisomy children. He has testified before the U.S. Senate that life begins with fertilization.

Professor G. Serlupi is the director of the Italian Institute that corresponds to the National Institutes of Health. He is a biochemist by trade, and a very fine gentleman.

The Rev. Padre Jan Visser is a Dutch priest who is a moral theologian in the Vatican.

The last member of the group besides H.W.J. and G.S.J. was Professor Robert J. White, director of Neurosurgery at Case Western Reserve and a Catholic layman, so to speak, but apparently very influential in the inner circles of the Catholic church.

The meeting was held in the Casina Pio IV. This is a small late Renaissance jewel right in the middle of the Vatican Gardens. Vatican City comprises a hundred and three acres, is bound on one side by St. Peters and its appendages, such as the Sistine Chapel and a large new auditorium where the pope has his public audiences, and then the old and new buildings that house the Vatican museums, on top of which is a belvedere where the pope may overlook the city of Rome. The rest of Vatican City is enclosed by walls so that the garden itself is probably of fifty acres, in the center of which stands the Casina Pio IV. It was built by Pope Pius IV as a summerhouse but has, of course, been much modernized in terms of plumbing and electricity. The meeting was held in a large seminar room, with a table that accommodated perhaps twenty seats within this summerhouse. The building was constructed in 1561. The seminar room had a barrel ceiling with a fresco dating from about that time. The Pontifical Academy of Sciences was founded in 1603 but apparently has recently taken on a new lease of life and its purpose is to inform the Vatican of progress in the mathematical, physical, and natural sciences, and in order to do this, organizes plenary sessions and work groups that eventuate in a document transmitted to the pope himself.

A sidelight of all this is that we were informed that as pontifical academicians, Georgeanna and I were entitled to be addressed by the titles of "Your Excellency" and that in the event of ecclesiastical procession, the pontifical academicians would march behind the cardinals and in front of the bishops. We were also informed that this distinction, if that's what it is, is a lifetime designation. We could hardly wait for some conclave that would allow us to get between Bishop Sullivan and the cardinals.

At the first meeting, Professor Chagas, who is a very distinguished and cultured gentleman, said that the meeting would be "free," and that "the walls have no ears." He also said that he would like to first discuss the scientific aspects of IVF, later touch on the social and economic implications, and then finally discuss the legal and moral aspects of it, although the real function of the academy was to produce a document that set forth the current scientific status of the program. He indicated that in order to develop the information, we would need to discuss cryopreservation of conceptuses, whether there were any abnormalities identified within IVF humans, etc., etc. He seemed resolved about the time period in which ensoulment occurs and, in fact, in the subsequent discussions there was no further discussion on this topic. It seemed to be assumed by him and by the clergy in attendance that human life began at fertilization.

H.W.J. and G.S.J. were the first called upon to present the state of the art. In view of the fact that in all of the communications there was no mention of any agenda, we had very few slides with us. Fortunately, I had brought along the slides of our results by year, the results by trial, and emphasized the inefficiency of human reproduction — specifically pointing out the selection process involved with the oocyte, on one hand, in which there is only one out of twenty oocytes in the ovary available for ovulation at the beginning of puberty, as well as pointing out that maybe as many as three out of four sperm were abnormal in one way or other, and that the union of sperm and egg in normal reproduction results in a pregnancy in any one cycle of only about 20 percent.

Professor Frydman then presented their results, also with very few slides because, like us, he had no idea what the agenda was. One of the special features of his presentation was their experience with the transvesicle and transvaginal routes for oocyte collection.

In the general discussion that followed, there was a great

deal of interest in knowing whether fertilization in vivo (specifically placing sperm and egg in the uterus) would work. They were surprised to find that it had been tried, even though very few times in our experience, and also René Frydman had tried it. They were unaware of the fact that Dr. Gary Hodgen (scientific director of the Jones Institute in Norfolk, Virginia) had tried it on some thirty-odd occasions in the monkey without success. Lejeune was particularly anxious to know why this was so, and one of the conclusions, which I am sure will be in the final written document, will be that more research might be expended on this particular process. I inquired if the Academy of Sciences was prepared to make grants in aid, but they said that this was outside of their possibility.

There was a good bit of discussion about experimentation on the conceptus. This was particularly relevant because J. P. II, in an address to a previous working party, had spoken about the undesirability of experiments on the conceptus. This provoked a discussion on the definition of 'experiment.' It was agreed that an experiment, in the sense that was of concern to the pope, implied its destruction by necessity of design during the course of the experiment. It specifically did not include such things as manipulation of the culture me-dium, for example, which might have, as an effect, the fail-ure of the conceptus to survive. Professor Chagas seemed to prefer the words 'observation' or 'modification,' saying that all these things were acceptable if the intent was to improve the state of the conceptus, even though in carrying out the procedure, the ultimate result might be the destruction of the conceptus.

It was pointed out by Professor Chagas that as we went

along, even though we were hopefully to confine our activities to the scientific aspect of IVF, the moral implications of the work were part of the discussion. At the end of the day, Chagas summed up and said it seemed clear that from the scientific or technical aspect that the technique was a viable, acceptable method and that its efficiency would be compared to that of normal reproduction.

The discussion the next day started off with a consideration of freezing and the preserving of conceptuses. Frydman explained the medical necessity for this, saying that it was medically unwise to transfer more than three fertilized eggs and that in order to preserve the conceptuses for later use, they had resorted to cryopreservation. Interestingly enough, Father Visser said that he felt that the scientist was under no obligation to use "extraordinary means" to preserve the conceptuses and that he regarded freezing as an "extraordinary means." He likened it to using "extraordinary means" to preserve life at the end of life. The other moral theologians present expressed considerable surprise, or perhaps "horror" is the more appropriate word, and the one that Father Visser would adopt. In discussing the matter of freezing, as the discussion went along, it seemed that the moral theologians were expressing concern about freezing not because of freezing per se and not because of preservation per se, but because the scientists present had said that the freezing process would inevitably destroy about 50 percent of the conceptuses. In other words, I thought that from an ethical point of view, they seemed to have no concern about preservation per se. In fact, if that were a method or an alternative to destroying conceptuses, they seemed to be for it. The discussion on freezing which went on for a considerable period of time and sort of ended without any clear resolution of what the eventual document from the discussion might say.

The discussion then turned to other technical aspects of IVF, such as the necessity to produce sperm by masturbation. It was interesting that they quoted Pius XII in 1949 as being against artificial insemination because it required masturbation. Much to my surprise, the moral theologians present made the point that no other pope had repeated this and that this question must now be reconsidered and certainly should not be an obstacle to a discussion of in vitro fertilization. Visser further pointed out that the important thing was the dignity of human procreation and that if this required masturbation, this must be an act of love to accomplish this particular objective (at lunchtime some of the moral theologians said that Visser was really a Dutchman and that the Dutchmen were really "way out there" on moral issues). Baumiller pointed out that Artificial Insemination by Husband (AIH), which required masturbation, was quite acceptable morally as far as he was concerned, and was widely practiced in Catholic hospitals.

There was a discussion of the definition of 'dignity.' Visser said that the Vatican did not mention dignity as a result of its deliberations, and as far as he is concerned dignity equated with human nature.

The final day of the meeting concerned out and out ethical issues in spite of the fact that they had been dragged in during the course of the earlier discussions. The lead-off man on the final day was Mons. Caffarra, who was considered by all the Romans present as being an arch-conservative. Caffarra listed several problems from his point of view. First was the fact that IVF separated intercourse from fecundation and interposed a third party in fecundation, in that the embryologist did the fecundation. Another point was the question of whether parents have the right to have children. He said that no human person has the right to have another person. Thirdly, he expressed concern about the fate of "spare" conceptuses. The final point was the fact that Humanae Vitae teaches conjugal love, and that IVF circumvented conjugal love.

There was a great deal of discussion about this latter point, and it went on and on and on. He was asked such questions as, "Suppose the embryologist who provided the opportunity for the sperm to fertilize the egg happened to be the husband?" "Why was there an interposition of a technician, and if there was an interposition, is this morally wrong?" "Was conjugal love synonymous with sexual intercourse?" etc., etc.

Baumiller, a Jesuit, said that at the time of Humanae Vitae, it was not possible for fecundation to occur without intercourse, but the world had moved on since then and that it was a time to have a new look at the problems.

Frydman pointed out that intercourse is not immediately related to fecundation anyway, but might be separated by as much as two or three days, and besides that, the husband did not fertilize the egg. He simply provided sperm for the egg to be fertilized, and that actually the embryologist was only facilitating the availability of the egg to meet the sperm; thus, the technician did not cause fertilization. Frydman also pointed out that there were many "embryologists" who are involved in reproduction, such as the obstetrician.

Caffarra was asked whether it was licit for individuals with nervous disorders, as for example, paraplegics, to have children, and he answered with an unequivocal "no." At the end of the discussion, I thought everybody had worked him over pretty good and that the only point he really could hold on to as a point of dogma was the matter of equating conjugal love with sexual intercourse, and that sexual intercourse had to be part of the process. I believe I am summarizing the attitude of the great majority of the discussants when I say that there was a general impression that this was an extremely narrow and old definition, and that conjugal love should indeed surpass this physical relationship in the human relation of marriage (at lunch Chagas said that the ultimate decision was going to be very interesting, that Caffarra had the right ear of the pope and that he himself, Chagas, had the left ear of the pope, and Chagas thought the pope himself was going to be the one who was going to have to make a decision).

After lunch on this same day, Chagas made a statement, a plea, really a very emotional discourse (which I am sorry I didn't have a recording of) in which he said that those who participate in IVF are really applying an act of love by taking an important step to preserve the family, that masturbation was an act of love for this purpose, and that the whole IVF program was an attempt to establish responsible parenthood. He pointed out his own infertility problem of seven years and what the birth of a child had meant to him, and that it created a new dimension of love. He said IVF is not only a technical question of morality in the philosophical sense, but was also a question of charity, and that those who were strict in the moral definition were not charitable. He ended up saying he made a plea not to condemn the method on a matter of principle. He said he was not necessarily asking for approval, but he was asking for at least silence. He said he was not a man of compromise, but a man of conciliation.

Baumiller said that on a pastoral level, when couples came to him to ask if it was wrong, he would ask them three questions: (1) Does it harm anyone? (2) Is it being done for a frivolous reason for simple convenience? (3) Is it medically necessary? (and if it had already been done, was the outcome good?). If a couple answered these questions in the way that he would anticipate, he would say they had committed no wrong.

The final discussion concerned the method of putting together the document that would result from the conference. All of the discussions were taped and I am not really sure how that was left. I think what will inevitably happen will be that Chagas, and probably Lejeune, will produce a document to circularize to members of the working group for review. I feel sure that all of this will take weeks, maybe even months, so that if the Vatican, i.e., the Pope, takes any action it will not be for a considerable period of time.

The working party did not have an audience with the pope. This was said to be quite unusual, as he usually did meet with the working parties. But he had been occupied by diplomats from Argentina and Chile who, in fact, in our seminar room one morning signed a treaty of peace between Argentina and Chile over some islands. The signature of the treaty, of course, would have to be ratified by the two governments, but they ejected us from our seminar room for the second morning of the discussion. Nevertheless, we had a coffee break with them. I had no idea who they were but there was a very handsome cardinal there speaking Spanish, so he may have been a cardinal from either one of the countries, or maybe he was the arbitrator or conciliator.

The whole experience was really quite unreal and I

think we can all be justly proud of the fact that Norfolk really turned out to be the main scientific input at the meeting, supplemented, of course, by René Frydman.

On a lighter but no less pleasant side, we had the opportunity to see Giulietta Micara (formerly a student in our lab) every day, and we shared with her the excitement of Friday, October 19, when her team was able to retrieve two eggs, both of which sounded a tad immature, but nevertheless they were the first eggs that had been secured in the program at the University of Rome. We had a chance to see Giulietta's laboratory, which is absolutely superb. The operating room is immediately next to the lab, but to date, they haven't been able to persuade the anesthesiologist to use the room because it doesn't have the necessary anesthetic gadgets in it; so, at the moment, they are working in the main O.R. which is a couple of floors away, but eventually this detail should be ironed out.

Georgeanna and I discussed the Vatican meeting on our flight home. We were impressed with the quality of debate, but astonished at Monsignor Caffarra's rigid attitude. Back in Norfolk, we immediately dispatched a letter to Professor Chagas to express our concerns, and this became the basis of a second meeting in Rome.

We received a standard letter from him thanking us for participating, but we never received the promised transcript. I doubt it was overlooked. Furthering my suspicions, the proceedings of our working party were not even on the published list of the Pontifical Academy, nor were the names of external consultants attending the meeting ever publicly listed with the single exception of Lejeune who was already a member.

Some years later, I asked my very good friend, the Jesuit Father Richard McCormick, if he remembered receiving an invitation to the same meeting. He had indeed, but had declined because he sensed that such working parties are expected to support a position already taken, and he suspected he might be in disagreement with that position as far as IVF was concerned. The Vatican is by no means free of politics. Father McCormick seems to have been proven correct, and Monsignor Caffarra had probably not made an idle boast but, going over the heads of the Academy, had persuaded the Magisterium to deny approval for IVF.

We received public confirmation in 1987 when the Vatican issued *"Instruction on Respect for Human Life in its Origin and on the Dignity of Procreation Replies to Certain Questions of the Day."* The document is better known by the first two words of its Latin title, *Donum Vitae.* Its purpose is set out in the foreword, as follows.

> *The Congregation for the Doctrine of the Faith has been approached by various Episcopal Conferences or individual Bishops, by theologians, doctors, and scientists, concerning biomedical techniques which make it possible to intervene in the initial phase of the life of a human being and in the very processes of procreating and their conformity with the principles of Catholic morality. The present Instruction, which is the result of wide consultation and in particular of a careful evaluation of the declarations made by Episcopates, does not intend to repeat all the Church's teaching on the dignity of human life as it originates and on procreation, but to offer, in the light of the previous teaching of the Magisterium, some specific replies to the main questions being asked in this*

regard. The exposition is arranged as follows: an introduc-
tion will recall the fundamental principles, of an anthropo-
logical and moral character, which are necessary for a proper
evaluation of the problems and for working out replies to
those questions; the first part will have as its subject respect
for the human being from the first moment of his or her ex-
istence; the second part will deal with the moral questions
raised by technical interventions on human procreation; the
third part will offer some orientations on the relationships
between moral law and civil law in terms of the respect due
to human embryos and fetuses and as regards the legitimacy
of techniques of artificial procreation.

Donum Vitae amounts to a detailed consideration of every
aspect of IVF and its associated technologies, including donor eggs, donor sperm, and surrogacy. It found them illicit on
Catholic moral grounds because they are outside the bonds of
conjugal love. The Instruction even stretches to other issues
that should not be contentious, such as artificial insemination
of a woman with her husband's sperm, which it found ille-
gitimate except when it facilitates the biological purpose of
sexual intercourse. For instance, it could be approved where
there was an abnormality of the genitalia that prevented normal deposition of sperm in the vagina.

Georgeanna was particularly incensed with *Donum Vitae*,
not only because it ignored the special meeting of experts at
the Vatican, but because it was naïve in its understanding of
physiology. She suspected that Vatican thinking was based on
popular belief about reproduction in farm animals instead of
what was known about the sexual physiology of humans. In
general, mammals only copulate when the female is in heat
or "estrus," which is when she is ovulating. Thus, coitus in

animals is strictly for procreation. In humans, however, there is no equivalent to estrus, because there are no external signs or changes of behavior when ovulation occurs, and consequently coitus occurs throughout the menstrual cycle, even at the least fertile time when a woman is actively menstruating. It is a matter of chance if shedding of an oocyte from the ovary and insemination during coitus occurs on the same day. The timing of ovulation in women mystified scientists until the early Twentieth Century, and for a long time it was suspected to occur during menstruation because of a false analogy with dogs, simply because they have uterine seepage at estrus. Besides, there is considerable variation in the timing of ovulation from cycle to cycle, and even between women.

Vatican pronouncements about human fertility have puzzled scientists since Pope Paul VI promulgated *Humanae Vitae* in 1968, the encyclical that forbade the birth control pill. Only natural family planning was permitted by abstaining from intercourse around the fertile time of mid-cycle, because it took advantage of a "faculty provided by nature." Thus, family size could be legitimately controlled, but only in a strict and quite ineffective way. In view of this history, it was too great a leap for the Vatican to consider procreation other than by sexual intercourse, or "conjugal love" as Caffarra described it.

Georgeanna wrote an open letter to the Pope in 1987 in which she brilliantly explained the anomaly.

> *I write in response to the Vatican 'Instruction on. .. Procreation' as a member of the large majority of the non-Roman Catholic religious community, Christian and Jewish. I write as a practicing gynecologist with a long record of investigative work in reproductive physiology and endocrinology. Perhaps even more importantly, I speak as a wife of 46*

years and the mother of three children with successful mar-
riages of 19, 15, and 14 years, respectively.

In 1984, my husband Dr. Howard W. Jones, Jr., and
I were invited to the Pontifical Academy of Science at the
Vatican for the purpose of explaining the technical and sci-
entific aspects of in vitro fertilization (IVF). We were de-
lighted to participate – as non-Catholics. We acknowledge
the Catholic Church as the largest organization for poten-
tial good in the world. We regarded the invitation as an ex-
pression of openness and genuine interest in the science of
reproduction.

Two years earlier we had participated in an IVF sym-
posium in Bari, Italy, at which the five major Italian uni-
versities had joined efforts to gain support for IVF from the
Vatican and from the Italian Ministry of Health. There we
had had the opportunity to discuss the ethical issues with
Monsignor Carlo Caffarra, one of the very conservative theo-
logians of the Vatican, and were amazed to learn that his
ethical objection to IVF had nothing to do with abortion,
which was the issue often raised in the United States. Rather,
the ethical problem, as he saw it, was that IVF "is outside
the bonds of conjugal love." My query was, "Do I under-
stand this that conjugal love is defined as intercourse?"
The answer was, "Yes." My response was then as it is now:
"Monsignor Caffarra, in this Twentieth Century you must
change your definition of conjugal love."

Pope Paul VI in the encyclical letter Humana Vitae
(1968) sought to enlarge the definition of conjugal love as
intercourse-for-reproduction by adding to the reproduc-
tive function the function of "unity." This is defined by one
theologian as "love union" and presumably means love or

bonding between couples, but it still makes the conjugal act and conjugal love inseparable. The unitive and procreative functions of the conjugal act are not permitted to be separated ("Instruction," Part 2B, Sec.4). Therefore, procreating without intercourse is illicit, and intercourse without the possibility of reproduction is illicit. In the Vatican document, the definition of conjugal love as intercourse unifies the ethical discussions of all topics related to reproduction. Contraception is prohibited because the act is no longer expressive of the procreative function. Artificial insemination and IVF are prohibited because the procreative function is not by the physical union of the husband and wife.

To me, this reasoning dehumanizes the definition of conjugal love – intercourse, if you will – by insisting that the physical and biological aspects of intercourse must be absolute. It is physiologically possible – and to me ethically permissible – in true conjugal love to separate the function of unity (I call it loving pleasure) from the procreative function, as in the postpartum lactation phase or in the menopause. It is certainly possible physiologically to separate the procreative function from intercourse either by artificial insemination or by IVF. But to me it is never ethical to separate the procreative function between two people from conjugal love. The strongest bonds of conjugal love are those between two loving individuals who are able to make responsible judgments in relation to family formation.

A definition which implies that intercourse is conjugal love, and that the sole function of intercourse is reproduction, does not differentiate between human beings and animals. It is unjust to burden Catholic couples with such a medieval definition. Conjugal love between two human beings should first be a bond of admiration, respect, and mutual interests that produces a lasting spiritual union usually consummated in the physical union of the conjugal act, intercourse.

Reproduction with family formation is surely one of the great pleasures and benefits resulting from the commitment made between two individuals joined in conjugal love and the act of intercourse is physically designed to assure successful culmination of the reproductive process. Because human reproduction is notoriously inefficient, the repetitiveness of the act must be ensured.

This link is made by enkephalin, a natural morphine secreted by the nervous system during intercourse, thereby rewarding us with a feeling of well-being and pleasure, and making intercourse addictive. If the process were otherwise, humanity would not have survived and flourished. This habit formation ensures us that intercourse will occur repetitively enough, in a species without a built-in ovulation signal, so that one intercourse during a month may be successfully timed, and often enough during a year so that one of the successfully timed ovulations will become fertile.

More importantly, in mature conjugal love, the physical act should be inseparable from the spiritual love and respect associated with one special individual in the marriage bond. The union of the pleasurable with the reproductive aspect of the conjugal act provides not only for successful reproduction but also for the stable family formation, which, in human beings as in the primates, is vital to the survival of the young.

The relative importance of these various aspects of intercourse changes as the individuals in a marriage grow older.

When age prevents reproduction and when childrearing is completed, intercourse still furnishes – without the possibility of reproduction – its natural function of pleasure. So it is that intercourse from a scientific point of view has not one function but three: (1) reproduction in the early years, (2) a bond to maintain the family formation as childrearing becomes important, and finally, (3) solace to the elderly.

This returns us to the Vatican viewpoint that intercourse is licit only for the purpose of reproduction and that every intercourse must be open to the possibility of reproduction. If one carries this viewpoint to its extreme conclusion, no sterile man or woman should have intercourse. This would include the postmenopausal woman who, presumably with her spouse, would be condemned to abstinence. As this is so obviously impossible and illogical, exceptions have been made to include "unity," for example, the menopause and known medical factors which interrupt fertility – excluding, of course, sterilization procedures. The necessity for the exceptions makes the fallacy of the premise apparent.

If then, the premise – that reproduction without intercourse is illicit or intercourse without reproduction is illicit – is incorrect, Vatican pronouncements against contraception should be reviewed and revised. Although the Vatican has precluded contraception because it induces a condition in which intercourse is not open for reproduction, yet it has made an exception for rhythm contraception. Such an exception is a scientific fallacy and a contrivance, for it is a well-established fact that intercourse after ovulation has occurred – which is the only effective rhythm method – is never open to reproduction. What is the difference between this form of contraception and taking a pill to ensure a cycle "never open to reproduction?" The answer is that the pill is "unnatural," therefore alien to God's laws. But certainly prohibiting intercourse in a marriage blessed by true conjugal love is unnatural.

The majority opinion of the theologians attending the symposium of the Pontifical Academy to investigate the scientific and ethical aspects of IVF was that basic IVF is an ethical consensus. Monsignor Caffarra was the sole dissenter from this consensus. His final statement was that accepting the IVF procedure as ethical would demand reconsideration of all past pronouncements on the subject of reproduction. The next theologian to speak pointed out that if accepting IVF as ethical meant that the Vatican needed to review and possibly revise all former pronouncements on reproduction, perhaps the time had arrived to do just that.

Those in attendance were to receive the final draft of the scientific and ethical discussions for their review and, if necessary, corrections prior to presentation of the document to the Pope for his enlightenment. But no such document was circulated. We therefore conclude that His Holiness is not acquainted with the scientific discussions by the physicians or the ethical judgments of the theologians convened for the express purpose of evaluating the scientific and ethical considerations of IVF. The recent Vatican publication therefore seems to make a mockery of this activity of the Pontifical Academy, which was established during the Renaissance to preclude another Galileo affair.

The Vatican would be well advised, as the twentieth century draws to close, to listen to the collective wisdom of the many dedicated and brilliant ethicists and scientists available within its walls. The Vatican should redefine conjugal

*love between human beings in terms that emphasize all-en-
compassing love instead of limiting it to sexual intercourse.
The Vatican should realize the scientific factualness — nat-
uralness if you will, God's law as I prefer — of the two-fold
function of intercourse reproduction, and pleasure, and the
changing importance of the two functions in the lives of two
individuals joined in conjugal love.*

*The pronouncements of natural law were expounded by
the early pagan philosophers; in the Judeo-Christian ethic,
the laws of nature were regarded as God's laws. We seek
to determine the scientific and logical explanation for all of
these wonderful and beautiful examples of God's laws. When
our investigations indicate either additional functions, such
as pleasure in intercourse, or additional therapeutic mea-
sures for correction of defects, such as IVF for the treatment
of infertility, we should accept these findings as further evidence of God's will for us to be inquisitive and rational. For
this is a world of reason that God in His mercy has provided
for us. When we know the fact, we must sometimes change
our definitions — and even our minds.*

The Vatican never replied to her letter, and I doubt if
Pope John Paul II ever saw it. It was, however, published in
Fertility News and when Professor Giuseppe Benagiano of the
University of Rome "La Sapienza" read it he was so impressed
that he arranged to visit us in Norfolk on his next trip to the
States.

At the Omni Hotel where he was staying, he invited us
to a conference in Rome, titled *The Evolution of the Meaning of
Sexual Intercourse in the Human.* He was anxious to explore the
issues she had raised and the rationale behind the Vatican's

insistence on the inseparable link between copulation and procreation. The professor hoped to raise money for the meeting, although it was only after a long search that the Ford Foundation agreed to sponsor it. We attended the meeting with our laboratory director, Lucinda Veeck, at the Palazzo Farnese in October 1992. The background and purposes of the meeting were elegantly outlined in Benagiano's introductory speech:

> *Central to our debate are the scientific discoveries of the twentieth century, which revealed fundamental differences in sexual behaviour between most higher animals, including non-human primates, and the human species. With very few exceptions, other female animals only permit mating at the time of ovulation, when they show associated anatomical and behavioural changes.*
>
> *By contrast, women will permit intercourse through the menstrual cycle, as well as through pregnancy, lactation, and after the menopause. Ovulation in the human is not only not associated with any external signs, but it is so well hidden that it was only in the 1930s that scientists first discovered when, in the menstrual cycle, a woman ovulates.*
>
> *It is therefore obvious that, for humans, intercourse is much more than simply the act of reproduction, and I believe that it is fair to state that the bonding power of sex within the couple has now been widely recognized by most religious and philosophical schools.*
>
> *There is however, a new aspect to this problem: Recent scientific advances have made it possible for couples to have sex without reproducing, or to reproduce without having had sex.*

Our new-found ability to separate the "bonding" from the "reproductive" aspects of sex challenges age-old ideas. For this reason, some have been reluctant to even discuss this topic in the fear that it may have disruptive consequences. Scientists, it has been argued, can easily go too far in their zealous manipulation of nature. Let me therefore reassure everyone here that we are not about to steer the meeting in any definite direction, or toward adopting any definite final position.

What I hope we will engage in here during the next two and a half days is the search for truth. As a scientist, I am only too (and painfully) aware of Claude Bernard's alleged definition of "scientific truth" as "an imaginary line dividing the error into two parts," the one containing already discovered errors and the one where errors still to be discovered lay hidden! In spite of this, I believe that we must proceed with our search for truth and this, I hope, is what we will be doing. Before mentioning the issue of the continuously changing shape of scientific truth, let me address openly the always present accusation that debating certain arguments means seeding doubt and that, in turn, may have "dangerous consequences." I take strong exception to this idea: it is the honest and public search for truth that must be the basis for every discussion.

Personally, I advocate a fundamental role for scientific research in the construction of bioethical concepts; at the same time, I also strongly believe that it is not up to the scientist, as such, to draw ethical conclusions from the biological facts he investigates.

A harmonious complementarity of roles requires that science provide data as objective as possible that philosophers and ethicists must accept (although certainly not critically), even when they contradict, as in the case of Galileo, traditional certainties and beliefs, while at the same time it is the task of ethicists to enunciate moral judgments. Their duty is to place the physical facts in a more global perspective, which takes the totality of problems into consideration.

This is not always easy because often we speak different languages, and the difference in language is a continuous source of misunderstanding and friction, when it is not a cause of frank hostility. It is in the nature of this meeting to be open to the danger of failing to communicate because words do mean different things to people involved in different disciplines. We must guard against this trap and patiently look for definitions we can all accept.

Bearing all of this in mind, I hope that we will be able to discuss the true significance of the unique features that the act of intercourse takes in the human. And here comes again the problem of scientific truth. During the course of this meeting, our Biologist and Anthropologist friends will point out the many differences in the process of ovulation and its consequences in the human female, when compared to practically all other animal females. This leads to a different pattern of intercourse for the human species.

Our friends will also tell us of recent discoveries which, to a certain extent, may at least in part destroy the clear-cut line we have drawn in the past between humans and non-humans.

Even given a certain degree of uncertainty, the question remains unaltered: what is the significance of these differences? Do they imply that the meaning of the act of intercourse is fundamentally different in the human? Does it therefore mean that, in the human, intercourse can be ethically accept-able even when it is stripped of its reproductive meaning, or, on the contrary, no such extrapolation can be drawn and, if so – why?

These and many others are, in my view, the questions that we shall pose to one another and then try to at least be-gin to provide answers.

To make the questions possible, we have decided to start the meeting with an overview of the most recent bio-anthro-pological information.

This will be followed by a review of the evolution of the meaning of the sexual act in the main cultures of our plan-et. When it comes to culture, we tend to be very egocentric in the sense of often ignoring, or almost, the views of other, equally important, cultural groups.

The meeting must, by force, focus on the act of inter-course if we want to carry it to some form of conclusion. We therefore have, on purpose, left out important topics such as homosexuality.

This does not mean that whenever you feel that it is nec-essary, you may not introduce other aspects of the problem.

I hope that in proceeding in this way we will be able to at least define the areas of broad agreement, those where some agreement is possible and those where opposite and irrecon-cilable positions will continue to exist.

My dream and my hope is to generate enough data and enough interest, so that others will enter this field and carry on the search for the true meanings of the act of sexual love.

The discussion affirmed what we already knew as gyne-cologists and biologists: the sexual behavior of *Homo sapiens* is different to lower animals. Copulation occurs more often than not when conception is impossible—during pregnancy, in amenorrhea, after the menopause, after removing the uterus or tubes, and at most times of the menstrual cycle. Consequently, although essential for the survival of the species, it has other roles and implications.

We hoped that the attendance of Cardinal Angelini, who occupied a position in the Vatican equivalent to the Secretary of Health, offered a channel of communication to the Vatican that might prompt a reconsideration of *Donum Vitae*. It was a faint-hearted hope. Carlo Caffarra, who still serves today as Archbishop of Bologna, was probably one of the main authors of the Instruction, and was created a cardinal in 2006 by another conservative, Pope Benedict XVI. *Donum Vitae* was issued under the aegis of the Congregation for the Doctrine of the Faith for whom the Pope, then just a cardinal, was a prefect.

The American Fertility Society created an ethics committee to consider the implications of the new technologies and felt it needed to respond after *Donum Vitae* appeared. We paid careful and respectful attention to the rationale of the document, but reaffirmed the society's advocacy of reproductive technologies.

Since then, IVF and its offshoots have spread around the world. Almost everywhere, the public has welcomed it, although there will probably always be minorities of various persuasions who reject it for theological or ideological reasons. In the light of advances in biomedicine, the Vatican updated its position on ART in 2008 by issuing, *"Instruction on Certain Bioethical Questions,"* otherwise known as *Dignitas Personae*.

The teaching of Donum Vitae remains completely valid, both with regard to the principles on which it is based and the moral evaluations which it expresses. However, new biomedical technologies which have been introduced in the critical area of human life and the family have given rise to further questions, in particular in the field of research on human embryos, the use of stem cells for therapeutic purposes, as well as in other areas of experimental medicine.

With regard to the treatment of infertility, new medical techniques must respect three fundamental goods: (a) the right to life and to physical integrity of every human being from conception to natural death; (b) the unity of marriage, which means reciprocal respect for the right within marriage to become a father or mother only together with the other spouse; (c) the specifically human values of sexuality which require "that the procreation of a human person be brought about as the fruit of the conjugal act specific to the love between spouses."

It is true that approximately a third of women who have recourse to artificial procreation succeed in having a baby. It should be recognized, however, that given the proportion between the total number of embryos produced and those eventually born, the number of embryos that do not produce children is extremely high. These losses are accepted by the practitioners of in vitro fertilization as the price to be paid for positive results. In reality, it is deeply disturbing that research in this area aims principally at obtaining better results in terms of the percentage of babies born to women who begin the process, but does not manifest a concrete interest in the right to life of each individual embryo.

It is often objected that the loss of embryos is, in the majority of cases, unintentional or that it happens truly against the will of the parents and physicians. They say that it is a question of risks which are not all that different from those in natural procreation; to seek to generate new life without running any risks would in practice mean

doing nothing to transmit it. It is true that not all the losses of em-
bryos in the process of in vitro fertilization have the same relation-
ship to the will of those involved in the procedure. It is also true that
in many cases the abandonment, destruction, and loss of embryos
are foreseen and willed.'

This theological review encompassed many other procedures, some of which had not even emerged at the time of
the earlier Instruction. These included many that are common today, such as intra-cytoplasmic sperm injection (ICSI),
cryopreservation of gametes and embryos, selective reduction
in multiple pregnancies, preimplantation genetic diagnosis
(PGD), hormonal contraception, gene therapy, and stem cell
therapy. They were condemned on the grounds that willful
destruction of embryos conflicts with the doctrine of ensoulment from the moment of fertilization, and the familiar narrow ruling about "conjugal love." There has been no change
in doctrine since our working party met all those years ago,
and it is unlikely to happen in the foreseeable future. But we
hope that Pope Francis will, in due course, reexamine the attitude of his church to assisted reproductive technologies.

9

THE QUESTION OF PERSONHOOD

Another challenge facing the coming of IVF to the Americas has been the continued efforts in several US states and in Costa Rica to legalize the recognition of personhood from the time of fertilization. The intention is not only to outlaw elective termination of ongoing pregnancies, but also to forbid the use of IVF on the grounds that it causes "abortion" of fertilized eggs transferred to patients, because many fail to produce a live birth.

A bill was introduced in the United States House of Representatives on January 5, 2013, to the effect that human life begins at fertilization. It was referred later the same month to the Subcommittee on the Constitution and Civil Justice. Congress has entertained such bills before, and people in knowledgeable positions predict that no further action will be taken. As far back as 1981, there was a congressional hearing for a similar bill that died.

In 2008, Colorado was the first state to attempt to legislate for the definition of personhood with the aim of recognizing full human rights from conception. It is not surprising that Colorado was ahead of the pack, because the principal advocacy group behind the movement, Personhood-USA, is headquartered there. The website for Personhood -USA has changed since 2012, but earlier it stated, *"We intend to build the support of at least two-thirds of the states in an effort to reaffirm personhood within the U.S. Constitution."* At the ballot, their efforts failed by the wide margin of 34 to 65. A second effort in 2010 also failed, this time by 29 to 70. A third attempt the next year failed even to solicit adequate signatures to appear on the ballot.

An alternate route through the legislative maze was attempted in Virginia in 2012. The bill stated, *"The life of each human being begins at conception."* In Virginia, it is possible to alter the constitution by legislation provided it is passed in both the House of Delegates and the Senate, and is signed by the Governor. In this case, the House vote on the bill on February 13 passed it by a majority of 64 to 34.

There was opposition to the bill led by the Virginia chapter of the pro-choice advocacy group, NARAL, and the National Infertility Association, RESOLVE. In response to their protests and testimonies, the Senate voted 24 to 14 to send the bill back to committee. When the legislature severely limited the time for oral testimony, advocacy groups decided to focus on the strategy that RESOLVE was making on behalf of patients by drawing attention to the impact the bill would have on medical care. One aspect that was particularly striking was the concern that ectopic pregnancies would put physicians in an untenable position, because saving the life of a pregnant woman by abortion at the cost of losing her unborn baby would put them at risk of prosecution. It would become murder to kill a fetus that was legally recognized as a person. The bill could not be recommitted again the same year, and it was not re-called for the following year's legislative session, so for all practical purposes it is probably dead.

This bill is an example of widespread efforts underway in more than twenty-five states across the country, including an upcoming Nebraska vote this year, in November 2014. If any should ever succeed, there would undoubtedly follow a legal battle to test whether state law contravenes the decision of the Supreme Court in Roe versus Wade (1973), which declared personhood starts at the gestational age of viability. Furthermore, IVF would be threatened by any state legislating for personhood from the moment of fertilization.

In October 2000, the Constitutional Chamber of the Supreme Court of Costa Rica handed down a ruling prohibiting the practice of IVF throughout the country. The case was Artavia Murillo et al. ("*In vitro* Fertilization") versus Costa Rica, Inter-Am. Ct. H.R. (ser. C) no. 257 (2012). The petition that led to this ruling argued that the practice of IVF was unconstitutional because Article 2 of the Costa Rican Constitution states that, *"life is inviolable."* Costa Rica is a signatory to the American Convention on Human Rights, a pan-American human rights treaty, in which it is stated that, *"Every person has the right to have his life respected. This right shall be protected by law and, in general, from the moment of conception. No one shall be arbitrarily deprived of his life."* The petition to the court claimed that the loss of human embryos during IVF is a voluntary deprivation of life.

When the Supreme Court accepted this argument, the only IVF center in the country, Instituto Costarricense de Infertilidad, was forced to close its operations. There is access to other types of infertility treatment which were never banned, although they are only provided in private settings for payment. Patients who required IVF treatment were either forced to look outside the country if they could afford it, or were left without recourse and forced to accept childlessness. Adoption is difficult in Costa Rica, as it is in most countries, and there is often discrimination against couples of lower socioeconomic status who apply to the register. Thus, the Supreme Court decision was a heavy blow to many couples who desperately hoped to become parents, and the sanctions against practicing IVF were comparable to the penalties for homicide.

Costa Rica is the only country in the world that has completely banned the practice of IVF. Since no more appeals are possible because the Supreme Court is the highest court in the land, the only resort is to bring a petition against the State of Costa Rica to the Inter-American Court of Human Rights for human rights violations. This process requires petitions to be screened first before the Inter-American Commission on Human Rights, which can decide either to accept or reject them based on whether due process has been followed. This requires an exhaustive effort to try every legal channel in the country where the alleged violation occurred, and such demanding procedures are likely to put off all but the most determined petitioners.

But in 2001 a group of ten couples jointly filed a petition which set in motion a twelve year battle to reinstate IVF in the country. The case passed the admission criteria in 2004, but it took six years for the Inter-American Court to notify the Government of Costa Rica that it would hear the case. Although the parties could have decided to settle early on and forego a trial, the patients chose not to negotiate because there was a possibility that a positive ruling would be a legal landmark that could help infertile couples in other countries where IVF needed defending. Countries that have submitted to the Inter-American Court's jurisdiction by signing on to the American Convention on Human Rights are listed online.

Through the long years of waiting, most of the original patients have lost their chances of conception owing to menopause or divorce; only a few managed to conceive by leaving their country to seek IVF treatment elsewhere. At least 140,000 couples are estimated to be left without access to their only means for establishing a pregnancy.

Finally, the case was heard at the Inter-American Court in San José in September of 2012. A couple of months later, the lengthy battle ended with the Court recognizing that Costa Rica was discriminating against infertile couples, and in blatant violation of their human rights. This was a historic ruling because it denied that embryos have personhood in law, and acknowledged the rights of patients to seek fertility treatment in their own country. This was the first time that an international court of human rights recognized infertility as a disease; it declared that member states must not create obstacles to treatment in either private or public healthcare systems.

The Court's decision is a beacon to urge societies around the world to care about infertility and protect patients' rights. Unfortunately for those living in Costa Rica, IVF services are unlikely to open for at least three more years because the Supreme Court has yet to acknowledge the Court's decision. The country's President has asked the Ministry of Health to propose legislation on the subject, but the Social Security System is only just beginning in 2014 to discuss how to implement the mandate.

At the same time, some religious groups, including the Catholic Conference of Bishops, are apparently in denial that the country has been found liable for human rights violations. Many lawmakers are being courted by them in the middle of an election year to table a restrictive law similar to the Italian legislation on assisted reproduction that banned embryo freezing and other procedures deemed to reduce their viability. Vitrification technology for unfertilized oocytes may appease the opposition, but would that be winning an argument only to lose the war?

Costa Rican patients deserve more sympathetic treatment from their government. They should be given access to all the treatment options that are taken for granted in many other countries, and anything less than that is a violation of their rights. In the meantime, we hear congratulatory remarks about progress towards achieving these goals, but one cannot avoid sadly reflecting on the fact that for at least another year, many couples will fall victim to this discrimination.

10
POSTSCRIPT FOR IVF

Before the advent of IVF, there was perhaps less than a 50-50 chance that a couple seeking help from a fertility specialist would successfully conceive. This statistic looked even more discouraging when cases of donor sperm for male infertility were excluded, because that remedy was always relatively effective. The revolution in reproductive technology over the past three decades has raised the chances of success for couples to rates approaching 100 per cent, but with two major provisos. On the one hand, they must be prepared to endure treatment until their goal of a viable pregnancy is reached, and that may require many attempts. On the other hand, they must be willing to avail themselves, if necessary, of donor gametes or even surrogacy arrangements.

Despite this upbeat appraisal, IVF and associated techniques called assisted reproductive technologies (ARTs) have led to some unexpected, unintended, and some say, problematic consequences for society at large.

The first is the dramatic change in the familial circumstances in which many of the children grow up. Not so long ago, the "nuclear family" was the norm and the only model that was socially acceptable. In its traditional definition, the family consisted of a mother and a father and children who had inherited half of their genome from each parent. This relationship, defined by marriage, breeding and rearing, has become blurred after gamete donation and surrogate motherhood were involved. In an extreme case, it is possible for a child to have no genetic relationship to either rearing parent and be gestated in the uterus of another woman. That child's circumstances growing up are not strictly comparable to those of conventional adoption after birth, because the new technology introduces additional relationships. It affords the parents an opportunity to have some choice about a gamete donor(s) and the commissioning of a surrogate for gestating their future baby, who in IVF surrogacy may be their genetic child. It must be said, however, that assisted conception is only responsible for a tiny portion of the changes affecting the traditional family model in the fertile population at large. Among those changes, single parenthood is perhaps the most dramatic. According to the American Community Survey, an average of six of every ten women in their twenties who gave birth in 2011 was unmarried, although the fraction varied with income, education, and race.

The second impact of technology is the elective and selective termination of conceptuses in multiple pregnancies. This procedure, often called "selective reduction," is peculiar to assisted reproduction in which ovarian stimulation is used, whether or not it involves IVF. Its prevalence is hard to estimate because there is no mandate requiring cases to be reported to local health officials. The implantation of supernumerary embryos results in intra-uterine crowding, which threatens the growth, health, and delivery of all the babies. Fortunately, the risks are diminishing by the trend towards milder stimulation and single embryo transfer in younger patients and, hence, there are fewer cases in which selective reduction is indicated.

The third impact arises from the selection of healthy embryos by preimplantation genetic diagnosis (PGD). This technology avoids the gestation of a baby that would otherwise have inherited mutations from one or both parents with seriously implications for health and lifespan. PGD is used for testing where two recessive genes are present, as in Tay-Sachs disease, or for a highly penetrating autosomal dominant gene, as in Huntington's disease, or for an X-linked gene, such as Duchenne muscular dystrophy. Families using PGD quite often have a first child who suffers or dies from the disease he/she inherited, while the younger siblings are healthy because they were selected as embryos for transfer to the mother. Despite the growing availability of this humane procedure, it remains controversial for anyone who regards the loss of embryos as destruction of human life. In my view, however, we must do our utmost to ensure healthy babies are delivered whenever possible.

The fourth societal impact would probably cause a greater division of opinion than the others if it was not so very rare and seldom discussed. It can be illustrated by a case presented to us by a couple who were both born deaf from an identifiable recessive mutation. They requested PGD to *positively* select for embryos so that their child would carry the same mutations and be born deaf like themselves, although otherwise healthy. But what would the children think later on about the decision made for them? We were faced with the dilemma of whether we should ever use PGD to perpetuate an abnormality. Most of us with good hearing find it difficult to imagine how socially isolating its absence can be, and despite the benefits of sign language, cochlear implants, and hopes based on stem cell research, it remains a grave disability. For the deaf couple, they feared that parental bonds to their children with normal hearing would be strained by a drift into mainstream society as they grew up. A similar argument has been made for PGD to select embryos with the autosomal dominant mutation for achondroplasia, although in this case the primary phenotype, dwarfism, is often accompanied by serious health problems. In an era when we strive to respect patient autonomy, these are dilemmas that challenge the compassion and conscience of medical providers and conflict with the Hippocratic Oath, *primum non nocere* (do no harm).

Finally, with my mind reflecting on history and my eye firmly set on the future, I believe that although IVF and other ARTs have come a long way since the breakthrough of Louise Brown's birth in the UK and Elizabeth Carr's in the USA, they can by no means be considered mature yet. All technologies are interim expedients, and it is our hope and expectation that current ones will be succeeded in due course by others that are even more effective, safe, and less expensive.

Regrettably, progress is not being made as rapidly as it might. One of the reasons is that it is obstructed by opponents who make arguments that may sound well-meaning but have the effect of denying people the chance to have one of the greatest joys in life—parenthood. We seldom hear nowadays the cruel accusation that people are made infertile as a punishment, but there is still the old repudiation of fertility treatment because it "encourages people to have more children in an already overcrowded world." And as I have described, there is continuing opposition based on an assumption that is not warranted by biology, namely, that personhood begins at fertilization. We acknowledge, however, that the care of human embryos presents fresh ethical challenges, although we must question if they are, in substance, so very different to the responsibilities of helping to bring new life into the world through other areas of OB/GYN?

Besides the technical and ethical issues of working in this field, there is the challenge of advancing knowledge through research to lay foundations for novel therapies in future. But fertility research has been one of the Cinderella fields of medicine. When surveys have been published regarding research priorities held by the public, pediatrics and cancer have consistently risen to top of the list, while fertility remains near the bottom. The percentage of medical research grants funded by the main federal agency, the NIH, has been falling, especially since sequestration in 2013, and scientists are aware that the funding level for reproduction by the NICHD compares unfavorably with most other institutes, and also excludes human embryo research. Big pharmaceutical companies have deserted contraception research, and few of the smaller firms are engaged in fertility drugs and diagnostics. The huge gap between the opportunities for progress and the resources needed cannot be met from the modest resources of charities.

Among the problems that pioneers faced, an important one remains unsolved to this day. We need to determine a way of identifying oocytes with the highest pregnancy potential, preferably using a non-invasive test, so that they are transferred to patients preferentially. Over the years, the appearance, chemistry, genetics, and physiology of the oocyte and its cumulus cells have been intensively studied for markers of their quality, but so far to no avail. When this vexing problem is overcome, it will be possible to transfer single embryos without seriously compromising the pregnancy rate. Instead of transferring two, three or even more embryos in the hope that one that will "take" (at the risk of them all implanting), one embryo will be transferred at a time, starting with a fresh one and followed in subsequent cycles by others, as necessary, drawn from the freezer bank. Perhaps no other advance would have as large and immediate impact in reducing multiple pregnancies. In this way, a single harvest of oocytes from a younger woman might raise the pregnancy rate to the 90 per cent range, while additionally lowering the costs of treatment.

Although widely practiced, PGD is still in its infancy. The scope has enormously expanded as a result of the Human Genome Project with its ongoing search for mutations responsible for inherited diseases. Advances in DNA amplification, DNA probe design, and gene chips are constantly being made to enable multiple mutations to be screened simultaneously in single embryonic cells. For example, a chip used by the Jewish Ashkenazi community for testing for Tay-Sachs disease also tests a number of other disease genes that are relatively common in that ethnic group. Whether testing is done pre-nuptially or by PGD in an IVF cycle, it avoids a pregnancy with a seriously affected baby. One day soon, it will surely be possible to screen for chromosome number and a host of single copy mutations, complex mutations, and copy number variants in a single test. The impact in reducing the burden of disease and early death are hard to comprehend, although screening will never, of course, eliminate fresh mutations.

Sometimes a major advance has a dampening effect on progress. This is true for ICSI which has revolutionized the treatment of male infertility, but at the cost of requiring female partners to undergo onerous IVF procedures and sidelining the study of spermatogenesis. Since ICSI has been proven safe and effective, there has been less investment in discovering how to boost the production of sperm, even though there is the highly desirable goal of conceiving by coitus instead of depending on the medicalization of reproduction.

While male fertility research is in the doldrums, no scientific efforts are being made with ectogenesis to my knowledge. That is a pity, because although it is horror fiction in *Brave New World*, there are some good reasons why the development of fetuses *in vitro* is a desirable technology, although not for the purposes that Aldous Huxley had in mind. The technical challenges will be colossal but, if they can be overcome, women who lack a uterus will no longer require human surrogacy, fetuses would not be exposed to risks from their mothers' choice of diet and addictions, and the abandonment of pregnancy to the laboratory by others would be the final liberation for women from their biology.

Gamete donation has been a stock in trade for fertility specialists since the 1950s, and has brought happiness to countless formerly childless homes. But, except where it is used to avoid inheriting a dreaded disease, it falls short of ideal and the natural desire to have children who are genetically related. The practice can create tensions about privacy, disclosure, and custody that occasionally explode and have to be settled in the courtroom. In the future, I predict that oocytes and sperm will be engineered *de novo* from blood, skin, or other somatic cells by reprogramming the genome. This was a mere dream until very recently, but researchers at Kyoto University have succeeded in generating germ cells from embryonic stem cells and, perhaps more significantly, from induced pluripotential stem cells derived from somatic cells in adult mice. After further manipulations, the cells were converted into gametes of either sex and, following fertilization *in vitro* and embryo transfer, surrogate mother mice delivered healthy pups. I see no reason why this triumphal feat of experimental biology cannot leap into the clinic one day, although it will need very extensive safety testing for children-to-be. Maybe the technology will go even further because mutations inherited by stem cells from the parent might be corrected in culture, even before the oocytes or sperm are formed. PGD would then become redundant.

Turning to the socioeconomics of fertility, it is surely time for infertility and its treatment to be recognized as an integral part of health care systems. In many European countries, IVF is responsible for 3-5 per cent of births. Denmark is a particularly good example because its system entitles everyone within a certain age range regardless of marital status or sexual orientation to three free cycles of IVF treatment. Public demand for these services has been so great that this generosity with public funds has had to be reined back, yet there remains a compassionate and generous attitude to people there with infertility.

In striking contrast, only about 1.5 per cent of all deliveries are from IVF in the United States. Health insurance for fertility treatment is only mandated in 15 out of 50 states, and just 35 per cent of patients seeking IVF have any sort of coverage, and to a degree that varies from state to state. Consequently, the distribution of services is uneven and unfair. In three states in which insurance is mandated, there are 50% more IVF services per capita than the national average, and that cannot be accounted for by differences in average age or the prevalence of infertility.

Recent history gives no cause for optimism because no more states have opted for mandation since 2001, and the *Affordable Care Act* of 2010 ("Obamacare") does not cover infertility. In a recent analysis of insurance company data, the extremely high costs of maternity care for twins and triplets could be significantly offset by providing infertility coverage for women up to the age of 40. In that scenario, infertility patients should seek IVF immediately, and preferably offered, where appropriate, single embryo transfer.

Forty years ago, pioneers in our field, most notably Bob Edwards, were scoffed at by public figures ranging from politicians to religious figures, and even by some Nobel Prize winners (whose pantheon he later joined). They declared that conception in a Petri dish could not be done. When the possibility of conception by IVF drew a little closer, they said it should not be done. More timid scientists and doctors would have cracked under the pressures which hurt them personally and professionally. But visionaries who persist eventually get their rewards, and in reproductive medicine it is the satisfaction of knowing that their efforts have helped millions of people to become happy parents.

Not so long ago, pregnancy in a woman without fallopian tubes, or fatherhood for a man with hardly any sperm, or the birth of a healthy child to parents carrying deadly mutations would have been regarded like biblical miracles. Today, however, they are taken for granted, and that is as it should be as progress rolls forward over one problem to the next. Conception by IVF is not yet the norm, and may never be, but it is sufficiently common that it scarcely raises an eyebrow today. Its history has passed through three stages that the German philosopher, Arthur Schopenhauer, said were natural progressions towards the revelation of truth.

First it is ridiculed.
Second it is violently opposed.
And third it is accepted as self-evident.

Glossary

amenorrhea. Suspension of normal menstrual cycles.

amniocentesis. A medical procedure in which a small amount of amniotic fluid surrounding the fetus is removed for prenatal genetic analysis.

aneuploidy. A chromosome (*q.v.*) complement in which there is an extra or missing chromosome(s).

blastomeres. The first (eight) cells produced by cleavage (*q.v.*) of a fertilized oocyte.

chromosome. The 46 chromosomes in a normal nucleus consist of linear DNA molecules encoding the genome and packaged in proteins.

cleavage (division). The first divisions of the fertilized oocyte by mitosis (*q.v.*).

conceptus. The product of fertilization at any stage from cleavage (*q.v.*) stages to fetus.

corpus luteum. A temporary endocrine organ forming in the ovary from the follicle (*q.v.*) after ovulation (*q.v.*) and which secretes progesterone and estrogen.

cryopreservation. The technology of freezing living cells and tissues.

culture medium. A physiological solution containing basic salts and usually supplemented with amino acids, fatty acids, micronutrients, proteins, and antibiotics.

cumulus granulosa cells. The halo of cells surrounding the oocyte (*q.v.*) while it grows inside the follicle (*q.v.*) and which is ejected with the oocyte during ovulation (*q.v.*).

Down syndrome. A clinical syndrome commonly arising from an error in meiosis (*q.v.*) when an additional chromosome #21 is incorporated, causing trisomy (*q.v.*) in the zygote and, hence, the fetus.

ectopic pregnancy. A pregnancy in which an embryo implants outside the uterus, and commonly in the fallopian tube (*q.v.*).

embryologist (clinical). IVF laboratory specialist who cares for patients' gametes (*q.v.*) and embryos.

endocrine gland. Glands that secrete hormones (e.g. thyroid, ovary, testis, etc.).

estrogen. The female sex steroid hormone which is mainly secreted in the menstrual cycle by the follicle (*q.v.*) and corpus luteum (*q.v.*). In pregnancy it is produced mainly by the placenta.

fallopian tube. A pair of tubes originating in the uterus (*q.v.*) which have open funnels near to the ovary where they can receive the ovulated oocyte(s) (*q.v.*).

follicle (ovarian). A spheroidal structure in the ovary that grows to the size of a grape at ovulation (*q.v.*). Each follicle nurses an oocyte (*q.v.*) and is responsible for estrogen (*q.v.*) secretion during the first half of the menstrual cycle.

FSH (follicle-stimulating hormone). A pituitary hormone which is required for follicle (*q.v.*) growth.

gamete. The oocyte or spermatozoon.

germ cell. The germinal cell of either sex before it matures to become an oocyte or spermatozoon.

germinal vesicle (nucleus). The nucleus of the growing oocyte before it matures.

gestation. Synonym for pregnancy.

gonadotropin. A general term for FSH, LH, and hCG (*q.v.*).

hCG (human chorionic gonadotropin). A hormone produced abundantly by the placenta and which is essential for maintaining secretion of progesterone from the corpus luteum (*q.v.*) early in pregnancy. hCG is the basis of the pregnancy test.

ICSI (intracytoplasmic sperm injection). A procedure performed in IVF laboratories in which a single sperm is injected into an oocyte to assist fertilization for men with low sperm counts/ quality.

laparoscopy. A technique for visualizing internal organs and spaces using a telescope ('key-hole surgery'). It has been superseded in IVF treatment by the transvaginal ultrasound (*q.v.*) procedure.

LH (luteinizing hormone). A pituitary hormone responsible for triggering ovulation (*q.v.*) and maintaining progesterone (*q.v.*) secretion from the corpus luteum (*q.v.*) during the second half of the menstrual cycle.

meiosis. A specialized nuclear division that occurs only during the maturation of oocytes and spermatozoa in which, (i) genes are recombined between pairs of homologous chromosomes (*q.v.*), and (ii) the number of chromosomes (*q.v.*) is halved to prepare for fertilization.

metaphase. A stage in the process of meiosis (*q.v.*) at which oocytes are arrested in development (at metaphase II) shortly before ovulation (*q.v.*) until fertilization.

mitosis. The process of cellular growth in which somatic cells divide to make identical copies.

oocyte. The female gamete (*q.v.*) or unfertilized egg.

ovulation. The process of ejecting the oocyte from a follicle, which is triggered by LH (*q.v.*).

parthenogenesis. The limited development that occurs when an oocyte (*q.v.*) is activated without fertilization by a sperm.

PGD (preimplantation genetic diagnosis). A procedure in an IVF laboratory in which one or more blastomeres (*q.v.*) are removed from an embryo for genetic analysis.

polar body. The first and second polar bodies are tiny cellular structures containing redundant DNA which are emitted from oocytes during meiosis (*q.v.*).

polycystic ovarian disease (PCO). An endocrine disorder of fertility and metabolism affecting follicle development.

progesterone. The steroid hormone from the corpus luteum (*q.v.*) dominating the second half of the menstrual cycle when it prepares the uterus (*q.v.*) for embryo implantation. The main source of progesterone during pregnancy is the placenta.

pronucleus. There are two pronuclei in fertilized eggs, one of maternal origin and the other paternal and each containing a half set of ('haploid') chromosomes (*q.v.*).

selective reduction. In multiple pregnancies that are risky to a mother and her fetuses, this surgical procedure is used to reduce the number of fetuses to one or two.

stem cells (including embryonic stem cells). Undifferentiated cells with enormous capacity for multiplication and which are canalized during development *in vivo* or *in vitro* to create specialized cell types.

stimulation (ovarian). The use of oral/ injected drugs to stimulate follicle growth for women with hypogonadism or in IVF treatment cycles.

surrogacy. A socially cooperative arrangement between a commissioning couple and a woman (surrogate) who will carry their pregnancy. Surrogacy may involve insemination of the surrogate for conception *in vivo* or during IVF in which the surrogate receives the couple's embryo(s) by transfer from the laboratory.

transfer/ replacement (intrauterine). The transfer of embryos conceived *in vitro* to the uterine cavity for gestation.

trisomy. A type of aneuploidy (*q.v.*) in which an extra chromosome is present in the nucleus of every cell (see Down syndrome).

ultrasound. A method involving sound waves instead of radiation for visualizing internal organs or a fetus *in utero*. In modern IVF practice, it is used to guide a needle to the ovaries for aspirating oocytes from follicles.

uterus. Anatomical term for womb.

vitrification. An alternative technology to cryopreservation (*q.v.*) which avoids ice formation for storing cells and tissues at low temperatures.

zygote. The fertilized egg (or ovum).

Bibliography of
Howard and Georgeanna Jones

Books (15)

Jones GS. *Management of Endocrine Disorders of Menstruation and Fertility*. American Lectures in Endocrinology. Springfield, IL, Charles C. Thomas, 1954.

Obstetrical and Gynecological Survey. Seegar Jones G: co-editor for Gynecological Endocrinology and Infertility; Jones HW Jr: co-editor for Gynecology. Baltimore, Williams & Wilkins, 1957-1989.

Novak ER, Jones GS. *Textbook of Gynecology*, 6th edition. Baltimore, Williams & Wilkins, 1961.

Jones HW Jr, Scott WW. *Hermaphroditism, Genital Anomalies and Related Endocrine Disorders*, 1st & 2nd editions. Baltimore, Williams & Wilkins, 1958, 1971.

Novak ER, Jones GS, Jones HW Jr. *Novak's Textbook of Gynecology*, 7-10th editions. Baltimore, Williams & Wilkins, 1965-1980. Translations in Chinese, French, Japanese, Portuguese & Spanish.

Jones HW Jr, Heller RH. *Pediatric and Adolescent Gynecology*, 1st & 2nd editions. Baltimore, Williams & Wilkins, 1966 & 1971 (also in Spanish).

Jones HW Jr, Rock JA. *Reparative and Constructive Surgery of the Female Generative Tract*. Baltimore, Williams & Wilkins, 1983.

Jones GS. *Dimensions for Growing Up*. Norfolk Planning Council, Norfolk, VA, 1983.

Jones HW Jr. *Ethical Considerations of the New Reproductive Technologies*. Ethics Committee of the American Fertility Society, Fertil Steril 46; Suppl 1, 1986.

Jones HW Jr, Jones GS, Hodgen GD, Rosenwaks Z. *In vitro Fertilization — Norfolk*. Baltimore, Williams & Wilkins, 1986.

Jones HW Jr, Jones GS, Ticknor WE. *Richard Wesley TeLinde*. Baltimore, Williams & Wilkins, 1986.

Jones HW Jr, Schrader C. *In vitro Fertilization and Other Assisted Reproduction*. Proceedings of the Fifth World Congress on *In vitro* Fertilization and Embryo Transfer (Norfolk, 1987). Ann NY Acad Sci 541; 1988.

Rock JA, Murphy A, Jones HW Jr. *Female Reproductive Surgery*. Baltimore, Williams & Wilkins, 1992.

Jones HW Jr, Jones GS. *War and Love*. Bloomington, IN, Xlibris, 2004.

Crockin SL, Jones HW Jr. *Legal Conceptions: The Evolving Law and Policy of Assisted Reproductive Technologies*. Baltimore. The Johns Hopkins University Press, 2009.

Jones HW Jr. *Personhood Revisited—Reproductive Technology, Bioethics, Religion and the Law*. Minneapolis, Langdon Street Press, 2013.

Book Chapters (108)

Jones HW Jr. Embryology and congenital malformations. In: Kimbrough RA (ed.): *Gynecology*, Philadelphia, JB Lippincott, 1965.

Jones HW Jr. Chromosomal considerations. Development of the genitalia. The basic forms of chromosomal aberrations (with Baramki TA). In: *Intra-Uterine Development*, Philadelphia, Lea & Febiger, 1968, pp 145, 253, 327.

Jones HW Jr: Intersexuality. In: Bartalos M (ed.): *Genetics in Medical Practice*. Philadelphia, JB Lippincott, 1968, p 191.

Jones HW Jr. Embryonic, anatomic, and physiologic considerations (female). In: Cooke RE (ed.): *The Biologic Basis for Pediatric Practice*. New York, McGraw-Hill, 1968, p 1082.

Jones HW Jr. Developmental disorders (female). In: Cooke RE (ed.): *The Biologic Basis of Pediatric Practice*. New York, McGraw-Hill, 1968, p 1087.

Jones HW Jr. Acquired disorders (female). In: Cooke RE (ed.): *The Biologic Basis of Pediatric Practice*. New York, McGraw-Hill, 1968, p 1093.

Jones HW Jr. Anomalies of the female genitalia. In: Alken CE (ed.): *Encyclopedia of Urology*. Berlin, Springer-Verlag, 1968, p 345.

Jones HW Jr. The intersex states. In: Alken CE et al (eds.): *Encyclopedia of Urology*. Berlin, Springer-Verlag, 1968, p 375.

Jones GS. Endocrine functions of the placenta. Development of the adrenal. In: Barnes AC, (ed.): *Intra-Uterine Development*. Philadelphia, Lea & Febiger, 1968, Chapters 3, 15.

Jones HW Jr, Baramki TA. Congenital anomalies. In: Behrman SJ, Kistner RW (eds.): *Progress in Infertility*, 1st and 2nd editions. Boston, Little, Brown, 1968, 1975, pp 63, 47.

Jones HW Jr. Operative treatment of the male transsexual. In: Green R, Money J, (eds.): *Transsexualism and Sex Reassignment*. Baltimore, Johns Hopkins, 1969, p 313.

Jones HW Jr. The diagnosis and treatment of congenital anomalies of the female generative tract. In: Moghissi KS (ed.): *Birth Defects and Fetal Development: Endocrine and Metabolic Factors*. Springfield, Charles C. Thomas, 1974.

Jones HW Jr, Andrews MC. Surgery for congenital anomalies of the uterus and vagina and for infertility. In: Ridley JH, TeLinde RW (eds.): *Gynecologic Surgery: Errors, Safeguards, Salvage*. Baltimore, Williams & Wilkins, 1974, p 202.

Jones HW Jr, Schirmer HKA, Hoopes PE. A sex conversion operation for males with transsexualism. In: Whitehead ED (ed.): *Current Operative Urology*. Hagerstown, Harper & Row, 1975. (Reprinted from Am J Obstet Gynecol 100:101, 1968).

Jones HW Jr, Jones GS. A summary of present cytogenetics and a vision of the future role of cytogenetics in obstetrics and gynecology. In: Eskes TKAB (ed.): *Aspects of Obstetrics Today*. Amsterdam, Exerpta Medica, 1975, p 45.

Jones HW Jr. Congenital anomalies. In: Caplan RM (ed.): *Advances in Obstetrics and Gynecology*. Baltimore, Williams & Wilkins, 1978, p 325.

Jones HW Jr. Problems of sex differentiation-surgical correction. In: Sumitt RL, Bergsma D (eds.): *Sex Differentiation and Chromosomal Abnormalities*. New York, Alan R Liss, 1978, p 63.

Rary JM, Cummings DK, Jones HW Jr, Rock JA, Julian CG. Cytogenetic and clinical notes on a girl with 46,X,I (yq) karyotype, H-Y antigen-negative, and a gonadoblastoma. In: Sumitt RL, Bergsma D (eds.): *Sex Differentiation and Chromosomal Abnormalities*. New York, Alan R Liss, 1978, p 97.

Baramki TA, Jones HW Jr. Rokitansky's syndrome. In: Hafez ESE, Evans TN (eds.): *The Human Vagina*. Amsterdam, Elsevier, 1978.

Jones HW Jr. Other factors associated with primary infertility. In: Pepperell RJ (ed.): *The Infertile Couple*. New York, Churchill Livingstone, 1980.

Jones HW Jr. Non-adrenal female pseudohermaphroditism. In: Josso N (ed.): *The Intersex Child*. Basel, S Karger, 1981, p 65.

Jones GS, Garcia J, Acosta A. Luteal phase evaluation in *in vitro* fertilization. In: Edwards RG, Purdy JM (eds.): *Human Conception in vitro*. London, Academic Press, 1982, p 297.

Jones HW Jr. The ethics of *in vitro* fertilization-1981. In: Edwards RG, Purdy JM (eds.): *Human Conception Control.* London, Academic Press, 1982, p 351.

Jones GS, Garcia JE, Acosta A, Wright GL Jr. The occurrence of luteal phase defects during a program for *in vitro* fertilization. In: van der Molen HJ (ed.): *Hormonal Factors in Fertility, Infertility and Contraception.* Amsterdam, Exerpta Medica, 1982, p 244.

Jones HW Jr. Reproductive impairment and the malformed uterus. Fertil Steril 36:137, 1981. Reprinted in: Wallace EE, Kempers RD (eds.): *Modern Trends in Infertility and Conception Control.* New York, Harper & Row, 1982, p 282.

Jones HW Jr. Sex chromosome abnormalities: intersex. In: Benso RC (ed.): *Current Obstetrics and Gynecologic Diagnosis and Treatment*, 4th edition. Los Altos, Lange Medical Publications, 1982, p 149.

Jones HW Jr, Jones GS, Andrews MC, Acosta A, Garcia J, Sandow B, Veeck L, Wilkes C, McDowell J, Wright G Jr. Aspects of the program for *in vitro* fertilization at Norfolk January 1, 1982 to August 8, 1982. In: *In vitro Fertilization and Embryo Transfer.* London, Academic Press, 1983, p 365.

Jones HW Jr. Factors influencing ovo-implantation and maintenance of pregnancy following embryo transfer. In: Beier HM, Lindner HR (eds.): *Fertilization of the Human Egg in vitro.* Berlin, Springer-Verlag, 1983, p 293.

Jones HW Jr. Metroplasty. In: Nichols DH, Anderson GW (eds.): *Clinical Problems, Injuries, and Complications of Gynecologic Surgery.* Baltimore, Williams & Wilkins, 1983, p 162.

Jones GS. The historic review of the clinical use of progesterone and progestin. In: Bardin CW, Milgrom E, Mauvais-Jarvis P (eds.): *Progesterone and Progestins*. New York, Raven Press, 1983, p 189.

Jones HW Jr, Acosta AA, Andrews MC, Garcia JE, Jones GS, Mantzavinos T, McDowell J, Sandow BA, Veeck L, Whibley TW, Wilkes CA, Wright GL Jr. What is a pregnancy? A question for programs of *in vitro* fertilization. Fertil Steril 40:728, 1983. Reprinted in: Bettocchi S, Carenza L (eds.): *Human In vitro Fertilization and Early Embryo Development*. Rome, CIC, 1984, p 175.

Jones HW Jr. Family formation by fertilization *in vitro*-now and then. In: Puett D (ed.): *Human Fertility, Health and Food*. United Nations, New York, 1984, p 3.

Jones HW Jr. *In vitro* fertilization. In: Garcia CR, Mastroianni L (eds.): *Current Therapy of Infertility 1984-1985*. Philadelphia, BC Decker, 1984, p 117.

Acosta AA, Garcia JE, Jones GS, Veeck L, Sandow BA, Jones HW Jr. Organization of an *in vitro* fertilization program. In: Harrison RF, Bonnar J (eds.): *Fertility and Sterility*. Lancaster, MTP Press, 1984, p 139.

Acosta AA, Garcia JE, Jones GS, Wright GL Jr. Corpus luteum function in patients with hMG/hCG induced ovulation for *in vitro* fertilization. In: Feichtinger W, Kemeter P (eds.): *Recent Progress in Human In vitro Fertilization*. Palermo, Italy, COFESE, 1984, p 57.

Jones GS. Luteal phase studies in stimulated and unstimulated aspirated cycles. In: Bettocchi S, Carenza L (eds.): *Human In vitro Fertilization and Early Embryo Development*. Rome, CIC, 1984, p 217.

Jones HW Jr. A program for human *in vitro* fertilization and embryo transfer. In: Osofsky H (ed.): *Advances in Clinical Obstetrics and Gynecology*. Baltimore, Williams & Wilkins, 1984, p 1.

Jones HW Jr. Surgical construction of an artificial vagina. In: Nyhus LM, Baker RJ (eds.): *Mastery of Surgery*. Baltimore, Williams & Wilkins, 1984, v 2, p 1227.

Jones HW Jr, Klingensmith GJ. Congenital adrenal hyperplasia. In: Shearman RP (ed.): *Clinical Reproductive Endocrinology*. London, Churchill Livingstone, 1985, p 362.

Jones HW Jr. Endocrine stimulation with various ratios of FSH and LH. In: Edwards RG, Purdy JM, Steptoe PC (eds.): *Implantation of the Human Embryo*. London, Academic Press, 1985, p 11.

Jones HW Jr. Factors affecting the luteal phase in IVF and ET programs. In: Testart J, Frydman R (eds.): *Human In vitro Fertilization*. Amsterdam, Elsevier, 1985, p 219.

Jones HW Jr. *In vitro* fertilization. In: Buttram VC, Reiter RC (eds.): *Surgical Treatment of the Infertile Female*. Baltimore, Williams & Wilkins, 1985, p 355.

Bernardus RE, Jones GS, Acosta A, Garcia J, Liu HC, Muasher S, Rosenwaks Z, van Uem J, Weinstein F, Jones HW Jr.

Stimulation with follicle stimulating hormone/human chorionic gonadotropin in an *in vitro* fertilization program. In: Rolland R (ed.): *Gamete Quality and Fertility Regulation.* Amsterdam, Elsevier, 1985, p 179.

Jones GS: The role of luteal support in a program for *in vitro* fertilization. In: Edwards RG, Purdy JM, Steptoe PC (eds.): *Implantation of the Human Embryo.* London, Academic Press, 1985, p 285.

Jones HW Jr. *In vitro* fertilization, 1981-1983. In: Besch PK (ed.): *Biochemistry of Reproductive Years.* Proceedings of Seventh Arnold O. Beckman Conference in Clinical History, Washington, DC, 1985, p 237.

Jones HW Jr. The selection of patients for *in vitro* fertilisation. In: Thompson W, Joyce DN (eds.): In vitro Fertilisation and Donor Insemination. London, Royal College of Obstetricians and Gynecologists, 1985, p 189.

Jones HW Jr. Indications for *in vitro* fertilization. In: Jones HW Jr, Jones GS, Hodgen GD, Rosenwaks Z (eds.): In vitro Fertilization-Norfolk. Baltimore, Williams & Wilkins, 1986, p 1.

Jones GS. Luteal phase in a program for *in vitro* fertilization In: Jones HW Jr, Jones GS, Hodgen GD, Rosenwaks Z (eds.): *In vitro Fertilization-Norfolk.* Baltimore, Williams and Wilkins, 1986, p 221.

Jones HW Jr. Overall results from *in vitro* fertilization. In: Jones HW Jr, Jones GS, Hodgen GD, Rosenwaks Z (eds.): *In vitro Fertilization-Norfolk.* Baltimore, Williams & Wilkins, 1986, p 288.

Jones HW Jr. Ethical issues in *in vitro* fertilization. In: Jones HW Jr, Jones GS, Hodgen GD, Rosenwaks Z (eds.): *In vitro Fertilization-Norfolk*. Baltimore, Williams & Wilkins, 1986, p 295.

Jones HW Jr. *In vitro* fertilization. In: Steinberger E, Frajese G (eds.): *Reproductive Medicine*. New York, Raven Press, 1986, p 363.

Jones GS, Muasher S, Acosta AA, Rosenwaks Z. The use of GnRH in an *in vitro* fertilization program. In: Bennink HJT (ed.): *Pulsatile GnRH 1985*. Haarlem, Netherlands, Ferring, 1986, p 199.

Jones HW Jr. The infertile couple. In: Fishel S, Symonds EM (eds.): *In vitro Fertilization*. Oxford, IRL Press, 1986, p 17.

Jones HW Jr. Status of basic external human fertilization. In: Slavkin HC (ed.): *Progress in Developmental Biology*, Part B. New York, Alan R Liss, 1986, p 275.

Jones HW Jr. Anomalies of the mullerian ducts. In: Rosenwaks Z, Benjamin F, Stone M (eds.): *Gynecology: Principles and Practice*. New York, Macmillan, 1987, p 147.

Jones HW Jr. Congenital anomalies of the uterus. In: Gondos B, Riddick D (eds.): *Pathology of Infertility*. New York, Thieme, 1987, p 29.

Jones HW Jr. Continuing pregnancy rates by number of concepti transferred. In: Feichtinger W, Kemeter P (eds.): *Future Aspects of Human in vitro Fertilization*. Berlin, Springer-Verlag, 1987, p 13.

Jones HW Jr. Oocyte recruitment with human menopausal gonadotropin (hMG) and follicle stimulating hormone (FSH). In: Naftolin F, DeCherney AH (eds.): *The Control of Follicle Development, Ovulation and Luteal Function: Lessons from in vitro Fertilization.* New York, Raven Press, 1987, p 211.

Jones HW Jr, Rock JA. Other factors associated with infertility: endometriosis externa, fibromyomata uteri. In: Pepperell RJ, Hudson B, Wood C (eds.): *The Infertile Couple,* 2nd edition. New York, Churchill Livingstone, 1987, p 181.

Jones HW Jr. Ovarian stimulation regimes with hMG and FSH for oocyte recovery. In: Ratnam SS et al (eds.): *In vitro Fertilization and Other Alternative Methods of Conception.* Parkridge, NJ, Parthenon, 1987, p 13.

Jones HW Jr. Bilateral chronic and symptomatic salpingitis: should hysterectomy be performed. In: Nichols DH, Anderson GW (eds.): *Clinical Problems, Injuries and Complications of Gynecologic Surgery,* 2d edition. Baltimore, Williams & Wilkins, 1988, p 72.

Jones HW Jr. *In vitro* fertilization. In: Behrman SJ et al (eds.): *Progress in Infertility,* 2nd edition. Boston, Little Brown, 1988, p 543.

Jones GS. Hormonal changes in perimenopause. In: Eskin BA (ed.): *The Menopause: Comprehensive Management,* 2nd edition. New York, Macmillan, 1988, p 237.

Jones HW Jr. Metroplasty. In: Nichols DH, Anderson GW (eds.): *Clinical Problems, Injuries, and Complications of Gynecologic Surgery,* 2nd edition. Baltimore, Williams & Wilkins, 1988, p 79.

Jones HW Jr. Preface. In: Jones HW Jr, Schrader C (eds.): *In vitro* Fertilization and Other Assisted Reproduction. *Proceedings of the Fifth World Congress on in vitro Fertilization and Embryo Transfer (Norfolk, 1987)*. Ann NY Acad Sci 541: xiii, 1988.

Jones HW Jr. Recent advances in *in vitro* fertilization (IVF). In: Izuka R, Semm K (eds.): *Human Reproduction: Current Status/ Future Prospect*. Berlin, Elsevier, 1988, p 65.

Jones HW Jr, Neuwirth RS. Abdominal metroplasty for a bicornuate uterus and a septate uterus. In: *OB GYN Illustrated* (pamphlet), LTI Medica, 1989.

Jones HW Jr, Rogers PAW. Results from *in vitro* fertilization. In: Wood C, Trounson A (eds.): *Clinical in vitro Fertilization*, 2nd edition. LTI Medica, 1989.

Jones HW Jr, Jones GS. Foreword. In: Acosta AA, Kruger TF (eds.): *Human Spermatozoa in Assisted Reproduction*. Baltimore, Williams and Wilkins, 1989.

Jones HW Jr. Ethical issues in surrogate motherhood: Commentary on ACOG Committee Opinion. In: *Women's Health Issues* 1(3), Opinion Number 88, Nov. 1990.

Jones HW Jr. Foreword. In: Miller RF, Brubaker BH (eds.): *Bioethics and the Beginnings of Life: An Anabaptist Perspective*. Herald Press, 1990.

Oehninger S, Acosta AA, Kruger TF, Veeck LL, Flood J, Jones HW Jr. Failure of fertilization in *in vitro* fertilization: the occult male factor. J *In Vitro* Fertil Embryo Trans 5:181, 1988. Reprinted in: *Yearbook of Infertility*. Year Book Medical Publishers, 1990.

Jones HW Jr. Ethical aspects of infertility and assisted reproduction. In: Insler V, Lunenfeld B (eds.): *Infertility: Male and
Female*. Churchill Livingstone, 1991.

Jones HW Jr. Historical perspective of congenital abnormalities of the female genital tract. Congenital malformations and
their treatment. In: *Clinical Practice of Gynecology*. Elsevier,
1991.

Jones HW Jr. Mullerian anomalies. In: *Gynecology*, 2nd edition.
Pergamon Publishing Company, 1991.

Jones HW Jr. Policy considerations for cryopreservation in *in
vitro* fertilization programs. In: *Issues in Reproductive Technology
I: An Anthology*. Garland Publishing, 1991.

Jones HW Jr, Rogers, PAW. Results from *in vitro* fertilization.
In: Wood C, Trounson A (eds.): *Clinical In vitro Fertilization*,
2nd edition. Springer-Verlag, 1991.

Jones HW Jr. Mullerian duct anomalies. In: Wallace EE, Zacur
HA (eds.): *Reproductive Medicine and Surgery*, Baltimore, 1991.

Jones HW. History of IVF. In: Insler V, Lunenfeld B. (eds.):
Infertility: Male and Female. Churchill Livingstone, London,
1991.

Jones HW Jr. Reconstruction of congenital uterovaginal anomalies. In: Rock JA, Murphy AA, Jones HW Jr (eds.): *Female
Reproductive Surgery*. Baltimore, Williams and Wilkins, 1992,
p 246.

Jones HW Jr. Surgical procedures for disorders of sexual development. In: Rock JA, Murphy AA, Jones HW Jr (eds.): *Female Reproductive Surgery*. Baltimore, Williams and Wilkins, 1992, p 287.

Jones HW Jr. *In vitro* assisted and other assisted reproductive technologies. In: Rock JA, Murphy AA, Jones HW Jr (eds.): *Female Reproductive Surgery*. Baltimore, Williams and Wilkins, 1992, p 379.

Jones HW Jr. Evolving aspects of reparative surgery. In: Thompson J, Rock JA (eds.): *TeLinde's Operative Gynecology*, 7th edition. JB Lippincott, 1992, p 739.

Jones HW Jr. Foreword. In: Jaffe R, Pierson RA, Abramowicz JS (eds.): *Imaging in Infertility and Reproductive Endocrinology*. JB Lippincott, 1993.

Jones HW Jr. Historical view of congenital malformations of the female genital tract. In: Verkauf BS (ed.): *Congenital Malformations and their Treatment*. Elsevier, 1993.

Toner JP, Singer J, Jones HW Jr. Uterine receptivity after ovarian stimulation for assisted reproduction. In: Giarnaroli L, Campana A, Trounson A (eds.): *Implantation in Mammals*.

Serono Symposia Publications, Raven Press, 1993.

Jones HW Jr. The many faces of morality. In: *Frontiers in Endocrinology: Perspectives on Assisted Reproduction*, Proceedings of VIIIth World Congress on *In vitro* Fertilization, Tokyo, Japan, 1994.

Jones HW Jr. Assisted reproduction. In: Chervenak FA, McCullough LB (eds.): *Ethical Dilemmas in Obstetrics*, 1994.

Stenchever MA, Jones HW Jr. Genetic disorders and sex chromosome abnormalities. In: DeCherney AH, Pernoll ML (eds.): *Current Obstetrics and Gynecologic Diagnosis and Treatment*, 8th edition. Appleton and Lange, 1994.

Jones HW Jr. Human development from fertilization to birth. In: Reich W (ed.): *Encyclopedia of Bioethics*. Macmillan Publishing Company, 1994.

Jones HW Jr. Bilateral chronic symptomatic salpingitis: should hysterectomy be performed? In: Nichols DH, DeLancey JO (eds.): *Clinical Problems, Injuries and Complications of Gynecologic and Obstetric Surgery*, 3rd edition. Baltimore, Williams and Wilkins, 1995.

Jones HW Jr. Mullerian duct anomalies. In: Wallach EE, Zacur HA (eds.): *Reproductive Medicine and Surgery*, 1st edition. Mosby, 1995.

Jones HW Jr. The Norfolk experience: How IVF came to the United States. In: *Pioneers in IVF*. Proceeding of a symposium, Oss, The Netherlands (1993). Parthenon Publishing, Lancaster UK, 1995.

Jones HW Jr. Foreword. In: *Principles and Practice of Assisted Reproduction*. WB Saunders and Company, 1995.

Jones, HW Jr. The many faces of morality - revisited. In: Aburumich A, Bernat E, Dohr G, Feichtinger W, et al (eds.): *IXth World Congress on in vitro Fertilization and Alternate Assisted Reproduction*. Monduzzi Editore, Bologna, Italy, 1995.

Jones HW Jr, Jones GS. A summary of present cytogenetics and a vision of the future role of cytogenetics in obstetrics and gynecology. In: Eskes TKAB (ed.): *Aspects of Obstetrics Today.* Amsterdam, Exerpta Medica, 1995, p 45.

Jones HW Jr. The history of *in vitro* fertilization. In: Keye WR, Chang J, Rebard RW, Soules MR (eds.): *Infertility: Evaluation and Treatment.* WB Saunders Company, 1995.

Jones HW Jr, Jones GS. Foreword. In: Adashi EY, Rock, JA, Rosenwaks Z (eds.): *Reproductive Endocrinology, Surgery and Technology.* Lippincott-Raven, 1996.

Jones, HW Jr. Foreword. In: Rock JA, Thompson JD (eds.): *TeLinde's Operative Gynecology,* 8th edition. Lippincott-Raven, 1997.

Jones HW Jr. Evolving aspects of reparative surgery. In: Rock JA, Thompson JD (eds.): *TeLinde's Operative Gynecology,* 8th edition. Lippincott-Raven, 1997.

Jones HW Jr, Jones GS. Luteal phase: physiology and pharmacotherapy. In: Diedrich K, Runnebaum R, Rabe T (eds.): *Manual on Assisted Reproduction.* Springer-Verlag, 1997.

Jones HW Jr. The USA experience. In: Brinsden PR (ed.): *A Textbook of in vitro Fertilization and Assisted Reproduction.* New York, Parthenon Publishing Group, 1999, p441.

Jones HW Jr. New reproductive technologies. In: Sureau C, Kohane-Shenfield F (eds.): *Balliere's Clinical Obstetrics and Gynecology.* London, Harcourt Publishing Co, 1999, p 473.

Jones HW Jr, McCormick RA, Crockin SL. Implantation in the human as viewed by canon law, civil law, and natural reason. In: D.D. Carson (ed.): *Embryo Implantation: Molecular, Cellular and Clinical Aspects*. New York, Springer-Verlag Inc., 1999, p 3.

Jones HW Jr, Jones GS. Luteal phase: physiology and pharmacotherapy. In: Rabe T, Diedrich K, Strowitzki T (eds.): *Manual on Assisted Reproduction*, 2nd updated edition. Springer-Verlag, Heidelberg, 2000, p 215.

Jones HW Jr. Regulation of assisted reproductive technology: The USA experience. In: Brinsden PR (ed.): *Textbook of In vitro Fertilization and Assisted Reproduction*, 3rd edition. Abingdon, UK, Taylor & Francis, 2005, p 661.

Jones HW Jr. The impact of assisted reproductive technology on gynecological surgery. In: Rock JA, Jones III, HW (eds.): *TeLinde's Operative Gynecology*, 10th edition. Philadelphia, Lippincott Williams & Wilkins, 2008, p 398.

Peer-Reviewed Publications/Invited Papers (527)

Jones HW Jr. Functional uterine bleeding with special reference to that associated with secretory endometrium. Am J Obstet Gynecol 35:64, 1938.

Jones HW Jr, Weil PG. The corpus luteum hormone in early pregnancy. JAMA 111:519, 1938.

Seegar, GE. Ovarian dysgerminoma. Arch Surg 37:697, 1938.

Gey GO, Seegar GE. Hellman LM. Production of gonadotropic substance (prolan) by placental cells in tissue culture. Science 88:306, 1938.

Jones HW Jr, Seegar GE. Ovarian tumors and uterine bleeding. Surgery 6:368, 1939.

Novak E, Jones HW Jr. Brenner tumors of the ovary. Am J Obstet Gynecol 38:872, 1939.

Jones HW Jr, Seegar GE. Mesonephroma of the ovary. Am J Obstet Gynecol 39:322, 1940.

Seegar GE. The histologic effect of progesterone on hyperplastic endometria. Am J Obstet Gynecol 39:469, 1940.

Seegar GE, Delfs E. Pregnandiol excretion following bilateral oophorectomy in early pregnancy. JAMA 115:1267, 1940.

Astwood EB, Jones GES. A simple method for the quantative determination of pregnandiol in human urine. Biol Chem 137:397, 1941.

Jones GES, TeLinde RW. The metabolism of progesterone in the hysterectomized woman. Am J Obstet Gynecol 41:682, 1941.

Jones GES, Astwood EB. The physiological significance of the estrogen: progesterone ratio on vaginal cornification in the rat. Endocrin 30:295, 1942.

Jones HW Jr, Jones GES. Mesonephroma of the ovary. Arch Path 33:18, 1942.

Jones HW Jr. Carcinoma of the cervix: clinical evaluation of radium dosage and supplementary roentgen irradiation based on a study of 915 cases. South Med J 35:959, 1942.

Jones GES, TeLinde RW. An evaluation of progesterone therapy in the treatment of endometrial hyperplasia. Bull Johns Hopkins Hosp 71:282, 1942.

Jones GES, Bucher NLR. Study of excretion of pituitary hormones in human urine. Endocrin 32:46, 1943.

Jones GES, Gey GO, Gey MK. Hormone production by placental cells maintained in continuous culture. Bull Johns Hopkins Hosp 72:26, 1943.

Jones HW Jr, Jones GES. Panhysterectomy versus irradiation for early cancer of the uterine cervix. JAMA 122:930, 1943.

Jones HW Jr, Neill W Jr. The treatment of carcinoma of the cervix during pregnancy. Am J Obstet Gynecol 48:447, 1944.

Jones GES, Delfs E, Stran HM. Chorionic gonadotropin and pregnanediol values in normal pregnancy. Bull Johns Hopkins Hosp 75:359, 1944.

Jones GES, TeLinde RW. The curability of granulosa-cell tumors. Am J Obstet Gynecol 50:691, 1945.

Jones GS, Everett HS. Arrhenoblastoma of the ovary, with a report of two cases. Am J Obstet Gynecol 52:614, 1946.

Jones HW Jr, Falor WH, Burbank CB. 1063 war wounds of the thorax and abdomen. Part II, pre- and post-operative care. J Mil Med Pacific, 1946.

Jones HW Jr, Falor WH, Burbank CB. 1063 war wounds of the thorax and abdomen. Part IV, wounds of the abdomen. J Mil Med Pacific, 1946.

Foote EC, Jones GES. An evaluation of the Hogben pregnancy test. Am J Obstet Gynecol 51:672, 1946.

Jones GES, Delfs E, Foote EC. The effect of thiouracil hypothyroidism on reproduction in the rat. Endocrin 38:337, 1946.

Falor WH, Jones HW Jr, Burbank CB. 165 acute combined wounds of the thorax and abdomen. Ohio St Med J 42:931, 1946.

Jones HW Jr, Falor WH, Burbank CB. 524 abdominal wounds on the western front. Bull Johns Hopkins Hosp 79:283, 1946.

Burbank CB, Falor WH, Jones HW Jr. Three hundred seventy-four acute war wounds of the thorax. Surgery 21:730, 1947.

Jones HW Jr, Cameron WR. Case-finding factors in cancer detection centers. JAMA 135:964, 1947.

Jones HW Jr. Testosterone in the treatment of advanced breast cancer. South Med J 41:4, 1948.

Delfs E, Jones GES. Some aspects of habitual abortion. South Med J 41:809, 1948.

Delfs E, Jones GES. Endocrine patterns in abortion. Obstet Gynecol Surv 3:680, 1948.

Jones GES, TeLinde RW. A survey of functional uterine bleeding with special reference to progesterone therapy. Am J Obstet Gynecol 57:854, 1949.

Guyton WL, Jones HW Jr. Pyogenic empyema with extension below with diaphragm. South Med J 4:359, 1949.

Jones GES. Some newer aspects of the management of infertility. JAMA 141:1123, 1949.

Jones HW. Carcinoma of the breast. Am J Surg 77:696, 1949.

Lewison EF, Levi JE, Jones GS, Jones HW Jr, Silberstein HE. Tracer studies of radioactive sodium estrone sulfate (S 35) in cases of advanced breast cancer. Cancer 4:537, 1950.

Jones HW Jr, Cameron WR. An appraisal of cancer detection centers. JAMA 143:228, 1950.

Ledogar JA, Jones HW Jr. The enzymatic dehydrogenation of estradiol to estrone. Science 112:536, 1950.

Jones GES, Delfs E. Endocrine patterns in term pregnancies following abortion. JAMA 146:1212, 1951.

Jones HW Jr. Non-puerperal inversion of the uterus. Am J Surg 81:492, 1951.

Jones HW Jr, Galvin GA, TeLinde RW. Intraepithelial carcinoma of the cervix and its clinical implications. Int Abstr Surg 92:521, 1951.Jones HW Jr: The detection of pelvic cancer. JAMA 146:1197, 1951.

Galvin GA, Jones HW Jr, TeLinde RW. Clinical relationship of carcinoma in situ and invasion of the cervix. JAMA 149:744, 1952.

Goldberg B, Wade OR, Jones HW Jr. Polysaccharide synthesis in frozen tissue sections as a histochemical method for phosphorylase. J Natl Cancer Inst 13:543, 1952.

Jones HW Jr, Wade R, Goldberg B. Phosphate liberation by endometrium in the presence of adenosinetriphosphate. Am J Obstet Gynecol 64:1118, 1952.

Jones HW Jr, Wade R, Goldberg B. Biochemical and histochemical alkaline glycerophosphatase in normal endometrium, endometrial hyperplasia, and adenocarcinoma. Am J Obstet Gynecol 64:1364, 1952.

Jones GES, Howard JE, Langford H: The use of cortisone in follicular phase disturbances. Fertil Steril 4:49, 1953.

Jones HW Jr, Jones GES: Double uterus as an etiological factor in repeated abortion: indications for surgical repair. Am J Obstet Gynecol 65:325, 1953.

Jones GS, Howard JE. The use of ACTH and cortisone therapy in obstetrics and gynecology. NY St J Med 53:2463, 1953.

Goldberg B, Jones HW Jr. Acid phosphatase in human female genital tract, a histochemical and biochemical study. Proc Soc Experimen Biol Med 83:45, 1953.

Jones HW Jr, Wade R. The effect of progesterone on phosphate release from adenosine triphosphate by rat liver homogenates. Science 118:103, 1953.

Jones GS. Medical aspects. Maryland St Med J 2:574, 1953.

Stran HJ, Jones GES. The filter paper electrophoretic identification of urinary chorionic gonadotropin. Bull Johns Hopkins Hosp 93:51, 1953.

TeLinde RW, Jones HW Jr, Galvin GA. What are the earliest endometrial changes to justify a diagnosis of endometrial cancer? Am J Obstet Gynecol 66:953, 1953.

Jones GS, Smith F: Treatment of the dysmenorrhea symptom complex: a preliminary report on the efficacy of a uterine "relaxing factor." Am J Obstet Gynecol 67, 628, 1954.

Stran HJ, Jones GES. Some properties of human urinary gonadotropins as elaborated by filter paper electrophoresis. Bull Johns Hopkins Hosp 95:162, 1954.

Klinefelter HF, Jones GS. Amenorrhea due to polycystic ovaries (Stein-Leventhal syndrome). JCEM 14:1247, 1954.

Lewison EF, Jones HW Jr, Doran WT Jr, Mandel B, Harrison C, Daniels R. Breast self-examination: educational and clinical effectiveness of the film. Maryland St Med J 3:123, 1954.

Wade R, Jones HW Jr. Inhibition of human endometrial adenosine triphosphatase by progesterone. Obstet Gynecol 3:608, 1954.

Goldberg B. Jones HW Jr. Some characteristics of the acid phosphatase of the human endometrium. Obstet Gynecol 4:426, 1954.

Jones GES, Jones HW Jr. Cortisone therapy in oligomenorrhea related to congenital adrenal hyperplasia. Studies on Fertil 6:140, 1954.

Jones HW Jr, Jones GES. The gynecological aspects of adrenal hyperplasia and allied disorders. Am J Obstet Gynecol 68:1330, 1954.

Galvin GA, Jones HW Jr, TeLinde RW. The significance of basal-cell hyperactivity in cervical biopsies. Am J Obstet Gynecol 70:808, 1955.

Jones HW Jr et al. Psychological aspects of the sexual orientation of the child with particular reference to the problem of intersexuality. J Pediatrics 47:771, 1955.

Wade R, Jones HW Jr. Effect of progesterone on oxidative phosphorylation. J Biol Chem 220:553, 1956.

Wade R, Jones HW Jr. Effect of progesterone on mitochondrial adenosinetriphosphatase. J Biol Chem 220:547, 1956.

Jones GES, Wade R, Jones HW Jr. Effect of progesterone on enzymatic systems. Proceedings of the Second World Congress on Fertility and Sterility, 1956, 373.

Goldberg B, Jones HW Jr. Acid phosphatase of the endometrium: histochemical demonstration in various normal and pathologic conditions. Obstet Gynecol 7:542, 1956.

Jones HW Jr, Delfs E, Jones GES. Reproductive difficulties in double uterus: the place of plastic reconstruction. Am J Obstet Gynecol 72:865, 1956.

Jones HW Jr, Galvin GA, TeLinde RW. Reexamination of biopsies taken prior to the development of invasive carcinoma of the cervix. Proceedings of the Third National Cancer Conference, 1957, 678.

Jones HW Jr. Hermaphroditism. Progress in Gynecology 3:35, 1957.

Jones HW Jr. Female hermaphroditism without virilization. Obstet Gynecol Surv 12:433, 1957.

TeLinde RW, Galvin GA, Jones HW Jr. Therapy of carcinoma in situ: implications from a study of its life history. Am J Obstet Gynecol 74:792, 1957.

Daughaday WE Jr (supported by a grant to Jones HW Jr). Apparatus for demarcating small areas in microprojection (aera, delineator). Lab Invest 6:558, 1957.

Swartz DP, Jones GES. Progesterone in anovulatory uterine bleeding. Fertil Steril 8:103, 1957.

Jones HW Jr. Amenorrhea and intersexuality. Maryland St Med J 7:104, 1958.

Wilkins L, Jones HW Jr. Masculinization of the female fetus. Obstet Gynecol 11:355, 1958.

Wilkins L, Jones HW Jr, Holman GH, Stempfel RS Jr. Masculinization of the female fetus associated with administration of oral and intramuscular progestins during gestation: non-adrenal female pseudohermpahroditism. JCEM 18:559, 1958.

Carey ML, Cian LC, Davis HJ, Boving B, Jones HW Jr. Experimental substitution of an isolate segment of ileum for the uterine tube. Obstet Gynecol 11:156, 1958.

Richter C, Jones GS, Biswanger L. Periodic phenomena and the thyroid. AMA Arch Neurol Psy 81:117, 1959.

Jones HW Jr, Goldberg B, Davis HJ, Burns BC Jr. Cellular changes in vaginal and buccal smears after radiation: an index of the radiocurability of carcinoma of the cervix. Am J Obstet Gynecol 78:1083, 1959.

Jones GES, Nalley WB. Amenorrhea: a review of etiology and treatment in 350 patients. Fertil Steril 10:461, 1959.

Jones HW Jr. Operations for congenital anomalies of the uterus and vagina. Clin Obstet Gynecol 2:1053, 1959.

Jones HW Jr, Wilkins L. The genital anomaly associated with prenatal exposure to progestogens. Fertil Steril 11:148, 1960.

Davis HJ, Jones HW Jr, Dickson RJ. The bioassay of host radiosensitivity. Cancer 12:358, 1960.

Jones HW Jr, McClelland ME. A study of delay in the treatment of pelvic cancer. Maryland St Med J 9:451, 1960.

Haddad HM, Jones HW Jr. Clitoral enlargement simulatin pseudohermaphroditism. AMA J Dise Child 99:282, 1960.

Lewison EF, Jones GS, Trimble FH, da Costa LL. Gigantomastia complicating pregnancy. Survey 110:215, 1960.

Fitz-William WG, Jones GS, Goldberg B. Cryostat techniques: methods for improving conservation and sectioning of tissue. Stain Tech 35:195, 1960.

Jones GES, Woodruff JD. Effect of a radiation opaque, water-soluble medium on the histopathology of the endometrium. Am J Obstet Gynecol 80:337, 1960.

Jones GS, Aziz Z, Urbina G. Clinical use of gonadotropins in conditions of ovarian insufficiency of various etiologies. Fertil Steril 12:217, 1961.

Jones HW Jr, Davis HJ. Radiation sensitivity testing for carcinoma of the cervix. Transactions of the Third World Congress of Obstet Gynecol 1961, 299.

Jones HW Jr, Wilkins L. Gynecological operations in 94 patients with intersexuality. Am J Obstet Gynecol 82:1142, 1961.

Johnston AW, Ferguson-Smith MA, Handmaker SD, Jones HW Jr, Jones GS. The triple-x syndrome: clinical, pathological, and chromosomal studies in three mentally retarded cases. Br Med J 2:1046, 1961.

Bergada C, Cleveland WW, Jones HW Jr, Wilkins L. Gonadal histology in patients with male pseudohermaphroditism and atypical gonadal dysgenesis: relation to theories of sex differentiation. Acta Endocrinol 40:493, 1962.

Bergada C, Cleveland WW, Jones HW Jr, Wilkins L. Variants of embryonic testicular dysgenesis: bilateral anorchia and the syndrome of rudimentary testes. Acta Endocrinol 40:521, 1962.

Moszkowski E, Woodruff DJ, Jones GES. The inadequate luteal phase. Am J Obstet Gynecol 83:363, 1962.

Jones HW Jr. Adrenogenital factors in abnormal menstruation. Bull St Barnabas Hosp, 1962, 60.

Jones GES, Jones HW Jr. Cortisone therapy in oligomenorrhea related to congenital adrenal hyperplasia. St Fertil 6:1940, 1962.

Jones GES, Acosta AA. Clinical use of pituitary reserve function test (SU 4885) in the diagnosis of amenorrhea. Am J Obstet Gynecol 84:701, 1962.

Jones GS, Pourmand K. An evaluation of etiologic factors and therapy in 555 private patients with primary infertility. Fertil Steril 13:398, 1962.

Jones GS, Moszkowski E. Alteracione en la fase lutea y su respuesta al tratamiento. El Dia Medico 34:872, 1962.

Jones GES, Turner D, Sarlos IJ, Barnes AC, Cohen R. The determination of urinary pregnanediol by gas liquid chromatography. Fertil Steril 13:544, 1962.

Jones HW Jr. Aplasia gonadal y sindrome triple X. El Dia Medico 34:880, 1962.

Jones HW Jr. Sub-committee for the study of pelvic cancer: reports. Maryland St Med J 11:18, 134, 187, 1962.

Goldberg B, Jones GES, Turner DA. Steroid3-β-ol dehydrogenase activity in some steroid-producing tumors. Am J Obstet Gynecol 8:1003, 1963.

Jones GS, Woodruff JD. Granulosa-cell-tumor diagnosis by urinary-estrogen assay. Obstet Gynecol 22:214, 1963.

Jones HW Jr. Sub-committee for the study of pelvic cancer: reports. Maryland St Med J 12:199, 455, 1963.

Jones HW Jr, Ferguson-Smith M, Heller R. The pathology and cytogenetics of gonadal agenesis. Am J Obstet Gynecol 87:578, 1963.

Heller RH, Jones HW Jr. Production of ovarian dysgenesis in the rat and human by busulphan.

Am J Obstet Gynecol 89:414, 1964.

Lau HL, Jones GS. The value of preparative thin-layer chromatography for the routine determination of pregnanediol. Am J Obstet Gynecol 90:132, 1964.

Jones HW Jr, McClelland ME. The changing clinical picture of carcinoma of cervix. Maryland St Med J 13:58, 1964.

Goldberg B, Jones GES, Borkowf HI. A histochemical study of substrate specificity for the steroid 3β-ol dehydrogenase and isomerase systems in human ovary and testis. J Histochem Cytochem 12:880, 1964.

Heller RH, Jones HW Jr. The production of ovarian dysgenesis in the rat by ethamoxytriphetol (MER-25). Am J Obstet Gynecol 90:264, 1964.

Jones HW Jr. Foreword. Am J Obstet Gynecol 90:984, 1964.

Ferguson-Smith MA, Alexander DS, Bowen P, Goodman RM, Kaufmann BN, Jones HW Jr, Heller RH. Clinical and cytogenetical studies in female gonadal dysgenesis and their bearing on the cause of Turner's syndrome. Cytogenet 3:355, 1964.

Jones HW Jr, Ferguson-Smith MA, Heller RH. Pathologic and cytogenetic findings in true hermaphroditism. Obstet Gynecol 25:435, 1965.

Jones HW Jr, Zourlas PA. Clinical, histologic, and cytogenetic findings in male hermaphroditism: male hermaphrodites with ambiguous or predominantly masculine external genitalia. Obstet Gynecol 25:597, 1965.

Zourlas PA, Jones HW Jr. Clinical, histologic, and cytogenetic findings in male hermaphroditism: male hermaphrodites with feminine external genitalia (testicular feminization). Obstet Gynecol 25:768, 1965.

Zourlas PA, Jones HW Jr. Clinical, histologic, and cytogenetic findings in male hermaphroditism: male hermaphrodites with asymmetrical gonadal differentiation (mixed gonadal dysgenesis). Obstet Gynecol 26:48, 1965.

Lau HL, Jones GS. Immunoassay of serum human chorionic gonadotropin by quantitative complement fixation and its comparison with the Delf's bioassay and two international standard preparations. Am J Obstet Gynecol 92:483, 1965.

Jones GS, Reuhsen M. Induction of ovulation with human gonadotropins and with clomiphene. Fertil Steril 16:461, 1965.

Jones HW Jr. Recent advances in gynecological cancer: ovary. Bull Sloan Hosp Women 11:122, 1965.

Jones HW Jr. Clinical significance of anomalies of the sex chromosomes. Am J Obstet Gynecol 93:335, 1965.

Messinger PS, Jones HW Jr. Indications for radical pelvic surgery. Clin Obstet Gynecol 8:611, 1965.

Novak ER, Goldberg B, Jones GS, O'Toole RV. Enzyme histochemistry of the menopausal ovary associated with normal and abnormal endometrium. Am J Obstet Gynecol 93:669, 1965.

Azoury RS, Jones, HW Jr. Cytogenetic findings in patients with congenital absence of the vagina. Am J Obstet Gynecol 94:178, 1966.

Jones HW Jr, Turner HH, Ferguson-Smith MA. Turner's syndrome and phenotype. Lancet 1:1155, 1966.

Uyeda CK, Davis HJ, Jones HW Jr. Nuclear protrusions and giant chromosome anomalies in cervical neoplasia. Acta Cytol 10:331, 1966.

Edwards RG, Donahue RP, Baramki TA, Jones HW Jr. Preliminary attempts to fertilize human oocytes matured in vitro. Am J Obstet Gynecol 96:192, 1966.

Davis HJ, Jones HW Jr. Population screening for cancer of the cervix with irrigation smears. Am J Obstet Gynecol 96:605, 1966.

Baramki TA, Jones HW Jr. Early premature menopause. Am J Obstet Gynecol 96:990, 1966.

Jones GS. Endocrine problems of the adolescent. Maryland St Med J 16:45, 1967.

Jones HW Jr. Congenital anomalies as a cause of primary amenorrhea. Maryland St Med J 16:49, 1967.

Jones GS, Goldberg B, Woodruff DJ. Enzyme histochemistry of a masculinizing arrhenoblastoma. Obstet Gynecol 29:328, 1967.

Katayama KP, Jones HW Jr. Chromosomes of atypical (adenomatous) hyperplasia and carcinoma of the endometrium. Am J Obstet Gynecol 97:978, 1967.

Jones GS. Diagnostic evaluation of patients with intersexuality. Ann NY Acad Sci 142:729, 1967.

Jones HW Jr. Gynecological surgery for patients with intersexuality: a report of 170 cases. Ann NY Acad Sci 142:747, 1967.

Rivarola MA, Saez JM, Jones HW Jr, Jones GS, Migeon CJ. The secretion of androgens by the normal, polycystic and neoplastic ovaries. Johns Hopkins Med J 121:82, 1967.

Arias-Bernal L, Jones HW Jr. An anencephalic male with XX sex chromosome complement. Am J Obstet Gynecol 99:877, 1967.

Jones HW Jr, Katayama KP, Stafl A, Davis HJ. Chromosomes of cervical atypia, carcinoma in situ, and epidermoid carcinoma of the cervix. Obstet Gynecol 30:790, 1967.

De Moraes-Ruehsen M, Jones GS. Premature ovarian failure. Fertil Steril 18:440, 1967.

Lopez JM, Migeon CJ, Jones GES. Hirsutism and evaluation of the dexamethasone suppression and chorionic gonadotropin stimulation test. Am J Obstet Gynecol 98:749, 1967.

Rivarola MA, Saez JM, Jones HW Jr, Jones GS, Migeon CJ. The secretion of androgens by the normal, polycystic and neoplastic ovaries. Johns Hopkins Med J 121:82, 1967.

Arias-Bernal L, Jones HW Jr. An anencephalic male with XX sex chromosome complement. Am J Obstet Gynecol 99:877, 1967.

Jones GS, de Moraes-Ruehsen M. Clomiphene citrate for improvement of ovarian function. Am J Obstet Gynecol 99:814, 1967.

Jones HW Jr, Katayama KP, Stafl A, Davis HJ. Chromosomes of cervical atypia, carcinoma in situ, and epidermoid carcinoma of the cervix. Obstet Gynecol 30:790, 1967.

Jones HW Jr, Schirmer HKA, Hoopes JE. A sex conversion operation for males with transsexualism. Am J Obstet Gynecol 100:101, 1968.

Katayama KP, Jones HW Jr. The chromosomes of normal and hyperplastic endometrium. Johns Hopkins Med J 122:84, 1968.

Jones GES, Goldberg B, Woodruff JD. Histochemistry as a guide for interpretation of cell function. Am J Obstet Gynecol 100:76, 1968.

Baggish MS, Woodruff JD, Tow SH, Jones HW Jr. Sex chromatin pattern in hydatidiform mole. Am J Obstet Gynecol 102:362, 1968.

Toews HA, Katayama KP, Jones HW Jr. Chromosomes of normal and neoplastic ovarian tissue. Obstet Gynecol 32:465, 1968.

Park IJ, Jones HW Jr. Glucose-6-phosphate dehydrogenase and the histogenesis of epidermoid carcinoma of the cervix. Am J Obstet Gynecol 102:106, 1968.

Jones GS. Menstrual dysfunction and oral conceptive drugs. JAMA 203-169, 1968.

Woodruff JD, Goldberg B, Jones GS. Enzymic histochemical reactions in two Krukenberg tumors associated with clinically different endocrine patterns. Am J Obstet Gynecol 100:405, 1968.

Arias-Bernal L, Jones HW Jr. Chromosomes of a malignant ovarian teratoma. Am J Obstet Gynecol 100:785, 1968.

Jones GS: Induction of ovulation. Ann Rev Med 19:351, 1968.

Poliak A, Jones GES, Goldberg B, Solomon D, Woodruff JD. Effect of human chorionic gonadotropin on postmenopausal women. Am J Obstet Gynecol 101-731, 1968.

Toews HA, Jones HW Jr. Cyclopia in association with D trisomy and gonadal agenesis. Am J Obstet Gynecol 102:53, 1968.

Jones HW Jr, Davis HJ, Frost JK, Park IJ, Salimi R, Tseng PY, Woodruff JD. The value of the assay of chromosomes in the diagnosis of cervical neoplasia. Am J Obstet Gynecol 102:624, 1968.

Jones GES, Goldberg G, Woodruff JD. Cell specific steroid inhibitions in histochemical steroid 3β-ol dehydrogenase activities in man. Histochem 14:131, 1968.

Lopez JM, Migeon CJ, Jones GS. Comparison of the estrogen feedback control mechanism between women with normal and polycystic ovaries. Am J Obstet Gynecol 103:555, 1969.

De Moraes-Ruehsen M, Jones GS, Burnett LS, Baramki TA. The aluteal cycle: a severe form of the luteal phase defect. Am J Obstet Gynecol 103:1059, 1969.

Jones GS, de Moraes-Ruehsen M, Johanson AJ, Raiti S, Blizzard RB: Elucidation of normal ovarian physiology by exogenous gonadotropin stimulation following steroid pituitary suppression. Fertil Steril 20:14, 1969.

Jones GS, de Moraes-Ruehsen M. A new syndrome of amenorrhea in association with hypergonadotropism and apparently normal ovarian follicular apparatus. Am J Obstet Gynecol 104:597, 1969

Jones HW Jr, Wheeless CR. Salvage of the reproductive potential of women with anomalous development of the mullerian ducts: 1868-1968-2068. Am J Obstet Gynecol 104:348, 1969.

Woodruff JD, Davis HJ, Jones HW Jr, Recio RG, Salimi R, Park IJ. Correlated investigative techniques of multiple anaplasias in the lower genital canal. Obstet Gynecol 33:609, 1969.

Davis HJ, Jones HW Jr. Cervical cancer control with irrigation smears. Obstet Gynecol Surv 24:927, 1969.

Jones HW Jr. Summary: detection and diagnosis of early cervical neoplasia: laboratory techniques. Obstet Gynecol Surv 24:993, 1969.

Jones HW Jr. Le traitement chirurgical des subjets masculins atteints de transsexualisme. Gyn Pratique 6:479, 1969.

Tseng PY, Jones HW Jr. Chromosome constitution of carcinoma of the endometrium. Obstet Gynecol 33:741, 1969.

Zourlas PA, Jones HW Jr. Stein-Leventhal syndrome with masculinizing ovarian tumors. Obstet Gynecol 34:861, 1969.

Salimi R, Jones, HW Jr. Chromosomes of adenocarcinoma of the cervix uteri with a ring and a minute marker chromosome. J Surg Oncol 2:17, 1970.

Lau HL, Ferraz E, Butler M, Jones GS. Comparison of a new covalent indicator-linked, immunochemical assay for human chorionic gonadotropin in serum with the Delf's bioassay. Johns Hopkins Med J 127:247, 1970.

Jones HW Jr, Woodruff JD, Davis HJ, Katayama KP, Salimi R, Park IJ, Tseng PY, Preston E. The evolution of chromosomal aneuploidy in cervical atypia, carcinoma in situ and invasive carcinoma of the uterine cervix. Johns Hopkins Med J 127:125, 1970.

Park IJ, Jones HW Jr. Familial male hermaphroditism with ambiguous external genitalia. Am J Obstet Gynecol 108:1197, 1970.

Park IJ, Jones HW Jr. A 48,XXXX female with mental retardation. Obstet Gynecol 35:248, 1970.

Barakat BY, Jones HW Jr. Gynecologic and cytogenetic aspects of gonadal agenesis and dysgenesis. Obstet Gynecol 36:368, 1970.

Jones GS, Madrigal-Castro V. Hormonal findings in association with abnormal corpus luteum function in the human: the luteal phase defect. Fertil Steril 21:1, 1970.

Neilson D, Jones GS, Woodruff JD. The innervation of the ovary. Obstet Gynecol Surv 25:889, 1970.

Verkauf BS, Jones HW Jr. Masculinization of the female genitalia in congenital adrenal hyperplasia. South Med J 63:634, 1970.

Jones GS, Maffezzoli RD, Strott CA, Ross GT, Kaplan G. Pathophysiology of reproductive failure after clomiphene-induced ovulation. Am J Obstet Gynecol 108(6):84, 1970.

Jones HW Jr, Verkauf BS, Lewis VG, Money J. The relevance of surgical, psychological, and endocrinological factors to the long-term end result of patients with congenital adrenal hyperplasia. Int J Gyn Obstet 8:398, 1970.

Jones HW Jr, Verkauf BS. Surgical treatment in congenital adrenal hyperplasia. Obstet Gynecol 36:1, 1970.

Park IJ, Jones HW Jr, Bias WB. True hermaphroditism with 46, XX/46, XY chromosome complement. Obstet Gynecol 36:377, 1970.

Jones HW Jr, Park IJ. A classification of special problems in sex differentiation. Birth Defects Orig Art Series 7:113, 1971.

Salimi R, Jones GS. The adreno-ovarian physiology in the rat treated with metopirone and corticosterone. Johns Hopkins Med J 129:332, 1971

Jones HW Jr, Verkauf BS. Congenital adrenal hyperplasia: age at menarche and related events at puberty. Am J Obstet Gynecol 109:292, 1971.

Barakat BY, Azoury RS, Jones HW Jr. Determination of fetal sex during the second trimester of pregnancy. Obstet Gynecol 37:134, 1971.

Bakarat BY, Heller RH, Jones HW Jr. Fetal quality control in pregnancies with high risk for genetic disorders. Fertil Steril 22:409, 1971.

Poliak A, Jones GS, Woodruff JD. The effect of human chorionic gonadotropin on castrated postmenopausal women. Am J Obstet Gynecol 109:555, 1971.

Jones HW Jr, McKusick VA, Harper PS, Wuu KD. George Otto Gey (1899-1970). Obstet Gynecol 38:945, 1971.

Sarria JA, Jones HW Jr. Implicaciones citogeneticas en la menopausai prematura. Rev Argentina Ginecol Obstet 2:171, 1971.

Spangler DB, Jones GS, Jones HW Jr. Infertility due to endometriosis. Am J Obstet Gynecol 209:850, 1971.

Jones HW Jr, Polacsek RA. The role of the medical journal in undergraduate education. J Reprod Med 7:120, 1971.

Jones GS. Women–the impact of advances in fertility control on their future. Fertil Steril 22:347, 1971.

De Moraes Ruehsen M, Blizzard RM, Garcia-Bunuel R, Jones GS. Autoimmunity and ovarian failure. Am J Obstet Gynecol 112:693, 1972.

Jones HW Jr, Money J, Meyer JK. An appraisal of the role of the gynecologist in the treatment of male transsexualism. Year Book Obstet Gynecol 1972, 276.

Katayama KP, Jones HW Jr: Chromosome studies of gynecologic malignancies by computer-oriented karyology. Clin Obstet Gynecol 15:236, 1972.

Katayama KP, Woodruff JD, Jones HW Jr. Chromosomes of condyloma acuminatum, Paget's disease, in situ carcinoma, invasive squamous cell carcinoma and malignant melanoma of the human vulva. Obstet Gynecol 39:346, 1972.

Wentz AC, Jones GS, Graeber J. Effect of infused prostaglandin F2α on hormonal levels during early pregnancy. Am J Obstet Gynecol 114:908, 1972.

Jones GS, Wentz AC. The effect of prostaglandin F2α infusion on corpus luteum function. Am J Obstet Gynecol 114:393, 1972.

Jones HW Jr, Mermut S. Familial occurrence of congenital absence of the vagina. Am J Obstet Gynecol 114:1100, 1972.

Park IJ, Pyeatte JC, Jones HW Jr, Woodruff JD. Gonadoblastoma in a true hermaphrodite with .46,XY genotype. Obstet Gynecol 40:466, 1972.

Park IJ, Jones HW Jr, Melhem RE. Nonadrenal familial female hermaphroditism. Am J Obstet Gynecol 112:930, 1972.

Jones HW Jr, Davis HJ, Frost JK. Opportunities and procedures for the early diagnosis of carcinoma of the cervix. Maryland St Med J 21:54, 1972.

Tremblay RR, Foley TP Jr, Corvol P, Park IJ, Kowarski A, Blizzard RM, Jones HW Jr, Migeon CJ. Plasma concentration of testosterone, dihydrotestosterone, testosterone-oestradiol binding globulin, and pituitary gonadotropins in the syndrome of male pseudo-hermaphroditism with testicular feminization. Acta Endocrin 70:331, 1972.

Park IJ, Johanson A, Jones HW Jr, Blizzard R. Special female hermaphroditism associated with multiple disorders. Obstet Gynecol 39:100, 1972.

Jones HW Jr. The surgical approach to problems of sexual identification. Med College VA Q 8:34, 1972.

Jones GS. Treatment of premenstrual gaseous abdominal distention. JAMA 220:1141, 1972.

Jones HW Jr. An anomaly of the external genitalia in female patients with exstrophy of the bladder. Am J Obstet Gynecol 117:748, 1973.

Mermut S, Katayama KP, Del Castillo R, Jones HW Jr. The effect of ultrasound on human chromosomes *in vitro*. Obstet Gynecol 41:4, 1973.

Wentz AC, Jones GS, Bledsoe T. Effects of PGF2α infusion on human cortisol biosynthesis. Prostaglandins 3:155, 1973.

Zourlas PA, Jones HW Jr. The gynecologic aspects of adrenal tumors. Obstet Gynecol 41:234, 1973.

Wentz AC, Jones GS. Intravenous prostaglandin F2α for induction of menses. Fertil Steril 24:569, 1973.

Jones GS. Luteal phase insufficiency. Clin Obstet Gynecol 16:255, 1973.

Jones HW Jr. Menometrorrhagia in patients with cervical dysplasia. JAMA 226:1126, 1973.

Wilks JW, Wentz AC, Jones GS. Prostaglandin F2α concentrations in the blood of women during normal menstrual cycles and dysmenorrhea. JCEM 37:469, 1973.

Wentz AC, Jones GS. Transient luteolytic effect of prostaglandin F2α in the human. Obstet Gynecol 42:172, 1973.

Jones GS. Treatment of single-partner sexual dysfunction. CMD 40:471, 1973.

Park IJ, Wentz AC, Jones HW Jr. The viability of fetal skin of abortuses induced by saline or prostaglandin. Am J Obstet Gynecol 115:274, 1973.

Park IJ, Heller RH, Jones HW Jr. Apparent pseudopuberty in a phenotypic female with a gonadal tumor. Am J Obstet Gynecol 119(5):661, 1974.

Jones HW Jr, Park IJ. Differential diagnosis in intersex conditions. Clin Plast Surg 1:223, 1974.

Aksel S, Wentz, Jones GS. Anovulatory infertility associated with adenocarcinoma and adenomatous hyperplasia of the endometrium. Obstet Gynecol 43:386, 1974.

Katayama KP, Park IJ, Heller RH, Barakat BY, Preston E, Jones HW Jr. Errors of prenatal cytogenetic diagnosis. Obstet Gynecol 44:693, 1974.

Aksel S, Jones GS: Etiology and treatment of dysfunctional uterine bleeding. Obstet Gynecol 44:1, 1974.

Umezaki C, Katayama KP, Jones HW Jr. Pregnancy rates after reconstructive surgery on the fallopian tubes. Obstet Gynecol 43:418, 1974.

Rary JM, Park IJ, Heller RH, Jones HW Jr, Baramki TA. Prenatal cytogenetic analysis of women with high risk for genetic disorders. J Hered 65:209, 1974.

Manuel M, Park IJ, Jones HW Jr. Prenatal sex determination by flourescent staining of cells for the presence of Y chromatin. Am J Obstet Gynecol 119:853, 1974.

Jones GS, Aksel S, Wentz AC. Serum progesterone values in the luteal phase defects: effect of chorionic gonadotropin. Obstet Gynecol 119:853, 1974.

Jones HW Jr. Surgical construction of female genitalia. Clin Plast Surg 1:255, 1974.

Keenan BS, Meyer WJ, Hadjian AJ, Jones HW Jr, Migeon CJ. Syndrome of androgen insensitivity in man: absence of 5 -dihydrotestosterone binding protein in fibroblasts. JCEM 38:1143, 1974.

Wentz AC, Jones GS, Andrews MC, King TM. Adrenal function during chronic danazol administration. Fertil Steril 26:1113, 1975.

Jones HW Jr, Jones GS. Amenorrhea (intermediate). Korean J Fertil Steril 2:5, 1975.

Jones HW Jr. Current status of uterine-suspension surgery. JAMA 234:332, 1975.

Wentz AC, Jones GS, Barnes HV. Diagnostic use of luteinizing hormone releasing hormone in primary amenorrhea. Obstet Gynecol 45:247, 1975.

Wentz AC, Rocco L, Jones GS. Effect of PGF2α in pseudopregnancy. Obstet Gynecol45:49, 1975.

Johnson JWS, Austin K, Jones GS, Davis GH, King TM. Efficacy of 17 alpha-hydroxyprogesterone caproate in the prevention of premature labor. N Eng J Med 293:675, 1975.

Park IJ, Aimakhu VE, Jones HW Jr. An etiologic and pathogenetic classification of male hermaphroditism. Am J Obstet Gynecol 123:505, 1975.

Wentz AC, Jones GS, Rocco L, Matthews RR. Gonadotropin response to luteinizing hormone releasing hormone administration in secondary amenorrhea and galactorrhea syndromes. Obstet Gynecol 45:256, 1975.

Wentz AC, Jones GS, Rocco L. Gonadotropin responses following luteinizing hormone releasing hormone administration in normal subjects. Obstet Gynecol 45:239, 1975.

Jones GS. The physiology of menstruation. Korean J Fertil Steril 2:1, 1975.

Manuel M, Katayama KP, Jones HW Jr. The age of occurrence of gonadal tumors in intersex patients with a Y chromosome. Am J Obstet Gynecol 124:293, 1976.

Amrhein MA, Meyer WM, Jones HW Jr, Migeon CJ. Androgen insensitivity in man: evidence for genetic heterogeneity. Proc Natl Acad Sci 73:891, 1976.

Park IJ, Burnett LS, Jones HW Jr, Migeon C, Blizzard RM. A case of male pseudohermaphroditism associated with elevated LH, normal FSH, and low testosterone possibly due to the secretion of an abnormal LH molecule. Acta Endocrin 83:173, 1976.

Jones GS. Culdoscopy. Clin Obstet Gynaecol 19:299, 1976.

Ju, KS, Park IJ, Jones HW Jr. The culturability of fibroblasts from the skin of abortuses after intra-amniotic instillation of urea or prostaglandin. Am J Obstet Gynecol 125:1155, 1976.

Wentz AC, White RI Jr, Migeon CJ, Hsu TH, Barnes HV, Jones GS. Differential ovarian and adrenal vein catheterization. Am J Obstet Gynecol 125:1000, 1976.

Wentz AC, Jones GS, Sapp KC. Effect of clomiphene citrate on gonadotropin responses to LRH administration in secondary amenorrhea and oligomenorrhea. Obstet Gynecol 47:677, 1976.

Wentz AC, Garcia SC, Klingensmith GJ, Migeon CJ, Jones GS. Gonadotropin output and response to LRH administration in congenital virilizing adrenal hyperplasia. JCEM 42:239, 1976.

Wentz AC, Jones GS, Sapp K. Gonadotropin output in menstrual dysfunction. Obstet Gynecol 47:309, 1976.

Aksel S, Wiebe RH, Tyson JE, Jones GS. Hormonal findings associated with aluteal cycles. Obstet Gynecol 4:598, 1976.

Wentz AC, Jones GS, Sapp KC. Investigation of danazol as a contraceptive agent. Contraception 13:619, 1976.

Neves-e-Castro M, Bruges e Savadra A, Vilhena MM, Jones HW Jr. Lateral communicating double uterus with unilateral vaginal obstruction. Am J Obstet Gynecol 125:865, 1976.

Jones GS. The luteal phase defect. Fertil Steril 27:351, 1976.

Aimakhu VE, Park IJ, Jones HW Jr. Male hermaphroditism with bilateral testes, well-formed mullerian structures, and 45,X chromosome complement. Obstet Gynecol 48:25s, 1976.

Katayama KP, Manuel M, Jones HW Jr, Jones GS. Methyltestostereone treatment of infertility associated with pelvic endometriosis. Fertil Steril 27:83, 1976.

Wentz AC, Jones GS. Office gynecology: managing dysmenorrhea. Postgrad Med 60:161, 1976.

Wentz AC, Gutai MP, Jones GS, Migeon CJ. Ovarian hyperthecosis in the adolescent patient. J Pediatr 88:488, 1976.

Ju KS, Park IJ, Jones HW Jr, Winn KJ. Prenatal sex determination by observation of the X-chromatin and the Y-chromatin of exfoliated amniotic fluid cells. Obstet Gynecol 47:287, 1976.

Wentz AC, Jones GS, Sapp KC, King TM. Progestational activity of Danazol in the human female subject. Am J Obstet Gynecol 126:378, 1976.

Wentz AC, Jones GS, Sapp K. Pulsatile gonadotropin output and response to luteinizing hormone releasing hormone (LRH) in primary amenorrhea. Obstet Gynecol 47:403, 1976.

Jones HW Jr, Garcia SC, Klingensmith GJ. Secondary surgical treatment of the masculinized external genitalia of patients with virilizing adrenal hyperplasia. Obstet Gynecol 48:73, 1976.

Babaknia A, Calfopoulos P, Jones HW Jr. The Stein-Leventhal syndrome and coincidental ovarian tumors. Obstet Gynecol 47:223, 1976.

Jones GS, Wentz AC. The structure and function of the corpus luteum. Clin Obstet Gynecol 3:43, 1976.

Jones HW Jr. Surgical procedure on oviduct to correct infertility. Fertil Steril 27:1219, 1976.

Jones HW Jr, Rock JA. Surgical treatment of female infertility. WHO Symposium on Advances in Fertility Regulation, Moscow, 1976.

Kunkel LM, Smith KD, Boyer SH, Borgaonkar DS, Wachtel SS, Miller OJ, Breg WR, Jones HW Jr, Rary JM. Analysis of human Y-chromosome-specific reiterated DNA in chromosome variants. Proc Natl Acad Sci 74:1245, 1977.

Jones GS. The clinical evaluation of ovulation and the luteal phase. J Reprod Med 18:139, 1977.

Rock JA, Jones HW Jr. The clinical management of the double uterus. Fertil Steril 28:798, 1977.

Jones GS, Wentz AC, Rosenwaks Z. Dynamic testing of hypothalamic-pituitary function in abnormalities of ovulation. Am J Obstet Gynecol 129:760, 1977.

Garcia JE, Cummings DK, Wentz AC, Jones HW Jr, Rary JM. A 5/X chromosomal translocation in a patient with premature menopause. J Hered 68:75, 1977.

Klingensmith GJ, Garcia SC, Jones HW Jr, Migeon, CJ, Blizzard RM. Glucocorticoid treatment of girls with congenital adrenal hyperplasia: effects on height, sexual maturation, and fertility. J Pediatr 90:996, 1977.

Jones HW Jr, Park IJ. Intersex. Clin Obstet Gynecol 20:545, 1977.

Garcia J, Jones HW Jr. The split thickness graft technique for vaginal agenesis. Obstet Gynecol 49:328, 1977.

Wentz AC, Schoemaker J, Jones GS, Sapp KC. Studies of pathophysiology in primary amenorrhea. Obstet Gynecol 50:129, 1977.

Garcia J, Jones GS, Wentz AC. The use of clomiphene citrate. Fertil Steril 28:707, 1977.

Krantz K, Millerick JD, Rosenwaks Z, Jones GS. Dysmenorrhea: quelling severe menstrual cramps. Patient Care 12:198, 1978.

Lau HL, Lawrence KW, Linkins SE, Jones GS. Early detection of human chorionic gonadotropin in urine by simple immunoassays. Am J Obstet Gyneco 132:691, 1978.

Rock JA, Katayama KP, Martin EJ, Woodruff JD, Jones HW Jr. Factors influencing the success of salpingostomy techniques for distal fimbrial obstruction. Obstet Gynecol 52:591, 1978.

Rary JM, Cummings D, Jones HW Jr. The fallibility of X-chromatin as a screening test for anomalies of the X chromosome. Obstet Gynecol 51:107, 1978.

Meyer WJ, Keenan BS, de Lacerda L, Park IJ, Jones HW Jr, Migeon CJ. Familial male pseudohermaphroditism with normal Leydig cell function at puberty. JCEM 46:593, 1978.

Jones HW Jr, Rock JA. On the reanastomosis of fallopian tubes after surgical sterilization. Fertil Steril 29:702, 1978.

Babaknia A, Rock JA, Jones HW Jr: Pregnancy success following abdominal myomectomy for infertility. Fertil Steril 30:644, 1978.

Wentz AC, Jones GS. Prognosis in primary amenorrhea. Fertil Steril 29:614, 1978.

Schoemaker J, Wentz AC, Jones GS, Dubin NH, Sapp KC. Stimulation of follicular growth with "pure" FSH in patients with anovulation and elevated LH levels. Obstet Gynecol 51:270, 1978.

Jones HW Jr, Park IF, Rock JA. Technique of surgical sex reassignment for micropenis and allied conditions. Am J Obstet Gynecol 132:870, 1978.

Jones HW Jr. Address of the honorary president: third world congress for cervical pathology and colposcopy. Obstet Gynecol Surv 34:786, 1979.

Rary JM, Cummings DK, Jones HW Jr, Rock JA. Assignment of the H-Y antigen gene to the short arm of chromosome Y. J Hered 70:78, 1979.

Rosenwaks Z, Lee PA, Jones GS, Migeon CJ, Wentz AC. An attenuated form of congenital virilizing adrenal hyperplasia. JCEM 49:335, 1979.

Katayama KP, Ju KS, Manuel M, Jones GS, Jones HW Jr. Computer analysis of etiology and pregnancy rate in 636 cases of primary infertility. Am J Obstet Gynecol 135:207, 1979.

Adashi EY, Rosenwaks Z, Lee PA, Migeon CJ. Endocrine features of an adrenal-like tumor of the ovary. JCEM 48:241, 1979.

Rosenwaks Z, Wentz AC, Jones GS, Urban MD, Lee PA, Migeon CJ, Parmley TH, Woodruff JD. Endometrial pathology and estrogens. Obstet Gynecol 53:403, 1979.

Adashi EY, Rock JA, Sapp KC, Martin EJ, Wentz AC, Jones GS. Gestational outcome of clomiphene-related conceptions. Fertil Steril 31:620, 1979.

Schweditsch MO, Dubin NH, Jones GS, Wentz AC. Hormonal considerations in early normal pregnancy and blighted ovum syndrome. Fertil Steril 31:252, 1979.

Jones GS. Hyperprolactinemia: an extension of the galactorrhea-amenorrhea syndrome. Obstet Gynecol Dig 21:21, 1979.

Jones HW Jr. A long look at the adrenogenital syndrome. Johns Hopkins Med J 145:143, 1979.

Rock JA, Rosenwaks Z, Adashi EY, Jones HW Jr, King TM. Microsurgery for tubal reconstruction following falope-ring sterilization in swine. J Microsurg 1:61, 1979.

Rock JA, Katayama KP, Martin EJ, Rock BM, Woodruff JD, Jones HW Jr. Pregnancy outcome following uterotubal implantation: a comparison of the reamer and sharp cornual wedge excision techniques. Fertil Steril 31:634, 1979.

Jones HW Jr, Rary JM, Rock JA, Cummings D. The role of the H-Y antigen in human sexual development. Johns Hopkins Med J 145:33, 1979.

Park IJ, Heller RH, Kaiser RM, Jones HW Jr. Spontaneous abortion after mid-trimester amniocentesis. Obstet Gynecol 53:190, 1979.

Jones HW Jr (panel moderator). Treatment of cervical intraepithelial neoplasia. Obstet Gynecol Surv 34:832, 1979.

Bibbins PE Jr, Wilds PL, Jones HW Jr, Rary JM. The crucial role of fetal age in amniotic fluid interpretation. VA Med 107:494, 1980.

Rock JA, Jones HW Jr. The double uterus associated with an obstructed hemivagina and ipsilateral renal agenesis. Am J Obstet Gynecol 138:339, 1980.

Jones HW Jr. The surgical correction of a double uterus. Pelv Surg 1:1, 1980.

Rock JA, Baramki TA, Jones HW Jr. A unilateral functioning uterine anlage in two patients with mullerian duct agenesis. Int J Gyn Obstet 18:99, 1980.

Cowan LD, Gordis L, Tonascia JA, Jones GS. Breast cancer incidence in women with a history of progesterone deficiency. Am J Epidemiol 114:209, 1981.

Rock JA, Guzick DS, Sengos C, Schweditsch M, Sapp KC, Jones HW Jr. The conservative surgical treatment of endometriosis: evaluation of pregnancy success with respect to the extent of disease as categorized using contemporary classification systems. Fertil Steril 35:131, 1981.

Garcia J, Jones GS, Acosta AA, WrightJr. Corpus luteum function after follicle aspiration for oocyte retrieval. Fertil Steril 3:565, 1981.

Adashi EY, Rock JA, Guzick D, Wentz AC, Jones GS, Jones HW Jr. Fertility following bilateral ovarian wedge resection: a critical analysis of 90 consecutive cases of the polycystic ovary syndrome. Fertil Steril 36:320, 1981.

Rosenwaks Z, Jones GS, Henzl MR, Dubin NH, Ghodgaokar RB, Hoffman S. Naproxen sodium, aspirin, and placebo in primary dysmenorrhea: reduction of pain and blood levels of prostaglandin F2-alpha metabolite. Am J Obstet Gynecol 40:592, 1981.

Jones HW Jr. Non-adrenal female pseudohermaphroditism. Pediatr Adolesc Endocrinol 8:6, 1981.

Garcia JE, Jones GS, WrightJr GL Prediction of the time of ovulation. Fertil Steril 35:308, 1981.

Bergquist CA, Rock JA, Jones HW Jr. Pregnancy outcome following treatment of intrauterine adhesions. Int J Fertil 26:107, 1981.

Begquist CA, Rock JA, Miller J, Guzick DS, Wentz AC, Jones GS. Artificial insemination with fresh donor sperm using the cervical cap technique: review of 278 cases. Obstet Gynecol 60:195, 1982.

Jones HW Jr. The ethics of *in vitro* fertilization-1982. Fertil Steril 37:146, 1982.

Jones HW Jr, Lee PA, Rock JA, Archer DF, Migeon CJ. A genetic male patient with 17a-hydroxylase deficiency. Obstet Gynecol 59:254, 1982.

Andrews MC, Jones HW Jr. Impaired reproductive performance of the unicornuate uterus: intrauterine growth retardation, infertility, and recurrent abortion in five cases. Am J Obstet Gynecol 144:173, 1982.

Lee PA, Rock JA, Brown TR, Fichman KM, Migeon CJ, Jones HW Jr. Leydig cell hypofunction resulting in male pseudohermaphroditism. Fertil Steril 37:675, 1982.

Rock JA, Zacur HA, Dlugi AM, Jones HW Jr, TeLinde RW. Pregnancy success following surgical correction of imperforate hymen and complete transverse vaginal septum. Obstet Gynecol 59:448, 1982.

Bibbins PE Jr, Anderson RL, Rary JM, Jones HW Jr. The prenatal diagnosis of the 48,XXYY syndrome. Prenat Diagn 2:123, 1982.

Jones HW Jr, Jones GS, Andrews MC, Acosta A, Bundren C, Garcia J, Sandow B, Veeck L, Wilkes C, Witmyer J, Wortham JE, Wright G. The program for *in vitro* fertilization at Norfolk. Fertil Steril 38:14, 1982.

Jones HW Jr, Acosta AA, Garcia JE. A technique for the aspiration of oocytes from human ovarian follicles. Fertil Steril 37:26, 1982.

Rock JA, Bergquist CA, Zacur HA, Parmley TH, Guzick DS, Jones HW Jr. Tubal anastomosis following unipolar cautery. Fertil Steril 37:613, 1982.

Channing CP, Liu CQ, Jones GS, Jones HW Jr. Decline of follicular oocyte maturation inhibitor coincident with maturation and achievement of fertilizability of oocytes recovered at midcycle of gonadotropin-treated women. Proc Natl Acad Sci 80:4184, 1983.

Jones HW Jr. Ethics of *in vitro* fertilization. Infertility 6:213, 1983.

Jones HW Jr. Financial aspects of a program of *in vitro* fertilization. Infertility 6:277, 1983.

Garcia JE, Jones GS, Acosta AA, Wright G. Human menopausal gonadotropin/human chorionic gonadotropin follicle maturation for oocyte aspiration. Phase 1, 1981. Fertil Steril 39:167, 1983.

Garcia JE, Jones GS, Acosta AA, Wright G. Human menopausal gonadotropin/human chorionic gonadotropin follicle maturation for oocyte maturation: Phase II, 1981. Fertil Steril 39:174, 1983.

Jones HW Jr, Acosta A, Andrews MC, Garcia JE, Jones GS,

Mantzavinos T, McDowell J, Sandow B, Veeck L, Whibley T, Wilkes C, Wright G. The importance of the follicular phase to success and failure in *in vitro* fertilization. Fertil Steril 40:317, 1983.

Veeck LL, Wortham JW, Witmyer J, Sandow BA, Acosta AA, Garcia JE, Jones GS, Jones HW Jr. Maturation and fertilization of morphologically immature human oocytes in a program of *in vitro* fertilization. Fertil Steril 39:594, 1983.

Jones HW Jr, Acosta AA, Garcia JE, Sandow BA, Veeck LL. On the transfer of conceptuses from oocytes fertilized *in vitro*. Fertil Steril 39:241, 1983.

Jones HW Jr. Results. Infertility 6:225, 1983.

Ferraretti AP, Garcia JE, Acosta AA, Jones GS. Serum luteinizing hormone during ovulation induction with human menopausal gonadotropin for *in vitro* fertilization in normally menstruating women. Fertil Steril 40:742, 1983.

Rock JA, Reeves LA, Retto H, Baramki TA, Zacur HA, Jones HW Jr. Success following vaginal creation for mullerian agenesis. Fertil Steril 39:809, 1983.

Jones HW Jr. Transfer. Infertility 6:183, 1983.

Mantzavinos T, Garcia JE, Jones HW Jr. Ultrasound measurement of ovarian follicles stimulated by human gonadotropins for oocyte recovery and *in vitro* fertilization. Fertil Steril 40:461, 1983.

Jones GS. The use of human menopausal gonadotropin for ovulation stimulation in patients for *in vitro* fertilization. Infertility 6:11, 1983.

Jones HW Jr. Variations on a theme. JAMA 250:2182, 1983.

Wortham JW, Veeck LL, Witmyer J, Jones HW Jr. Vital initiation of pregnancy (VIP) using human menopausal gonadotropin and human chorionic gonadotropin ovulation induction: Phase I-1981. Fertil Steril 39:785, 1983.

Wortham JW, Veeck LL, Witmyer J, Sandow BA, Jones HW Jr. Vital initiation of pregnancy (VIP) using human menopausal gonadotropin and human chorionic gonadotropin ovulation induction: Phase II-1981. Fertil Steril 40:170, 1983.

Jones HW Jr, Acosta AA, Andrews MC, Garcia JE, Jones GS, Mantzavinos T, McDowell J, Sandow BA, Veeck L, Whibley TW, Wilkes CA, Wright Jr GL. What is a pregnancy? A question for programs of *in vitro* fertilization. Fertil Steril 40:728, 1983.

Garcia JE, Acosta AA, Hsiu JG, Jones HW Jr. Advanced endometrial maturation after ovulation induction with human menopausal gonadotropin/human chorionic gonadotropin for *in vitro* fertilization. Fertil Steril 41:31, 1984.

Muasher SJ, Wilkes C, Garcia JE, Rosenwaks Z, Jones HW Jr. Benefits and risks of multiple transfer with *in vitro* fertilization. Lancet 1:570, 1984.

Rock JA, Schlaff WD, Zacur HA, Jones HW Jr. The clinical management of congenital absence of the uterine cervix. Int J Gyn Obstet 22:231, 1984.

Acosta AA, Jones GS, Garcia JE, Sandow B, Veeck L, Mantzavinos T. Correlation of human menopausal gonadotropin/human chorionic gonadotropin stimulation and oocyte quality in an *in vitro* fertilization program. Fertil Steril 41:196, 1984.

Muasher SJ, Garcia JE, Jones HW Jr. Experience with diethylstilbestrol-exposed infertile women in a program of *in vitro* fertilization. Fertil Steril 42:20, 1984.

Garcia J, Acosta A, Andrews MC, Jones G, Jones HW Jr, Mantzavinos T, Mayer J, McDowell J, Sandow B, Veeck L, Wilkes C, Wright G. *In vitro* fertilization in Norfolk, Virginia, 1980-1983. J *In vitro* Fert 1:24, 1984.

Channing CP, Tanabe K, Jones GS, Jones HW Jr, Lebeche P. Inhibin activity of preovulatory follicles of gonadotropin-treated and untreated women. Fertil Steril 42:243, 1984.

Muasher S, Acosta AA, Garcia JE, Jones GS, Jones HW Jr. Luteal phase serum estradiol and progesterone in *in vitro* fertilization. Fertil Steril 41:838, 1984.

Mishell DRJr, Fisher HW, Haynes PJ, Jones GS, Smith RP. Menorrhagia: a symposium. J Reprod Me 29:763s, 1984.

Jones GS, Garcia JE, Rosenwaks Z. The role of pituitary gonadotropins in follicular stimulation and oocyte maturation in the human. JCEM 59:178, 1984.

Jones HW Jr, Acosta AA, Andrews MC, Garcia JE, Jones GS, Mayer J, McDowell J, Rosenwaks Z, Sandow BA, Veeck LL, Wilkes CA. Three years of *in vitro* fertilization at Norfolk. Fertil Steril 42:826, 1984.

Jones GS. Update on *in vitro* fertilization. Endocrin Rev 5:62, 1984.

Rock JA, Jones HW Jr. Vaginal forms for dilatation and/or to maintain vaginal patency. Fertil Steril 42:187, 1984.

Muasher SJ, Acosta AA, Garcia JE, Rosenwaks Z, Jones HW Jr. Wedge metroplasty for the septate uterus: an update. Fertil Steril 42:515, 1984.

McDowell JS, Veeck LL, Jones HW Jr. Analysis of human spermatozoa before and after processing for *in vitro* fertilization. JIVF 2:23, 1985.

Given JE, Jones GS, McMillen DL. A comparison of personality characteristics between *in vitro* fertilization patients and other infertile patients. JIVF 2:49, 1985.

Simonetti S, Veeck LL, Jones HW Jr. Correlation of follicular fluid volume with oocyte morphology from follicles stimulated by human menopausal gonadotropin. Fertil Steril 44:177, 1985.

Jones HW Jr: Embryo transfer. Ann NY Acad Sci 442:375, 1985.

Jones HW Jr. Ethics of *in vitro* fertilization: 1984. Ann NY Acad Sci 442:577, 1985.

Rock JA, Wentz AC, Cole KA, Kimball HW Jr, Zacur HA, Early SA, Jones GS. Fetal malformations following progesterone therapy during pregnancy: a preliminary report. Fertil Steril 44:17, 1985.

Edwards RG, Seppala M, Johnston WI, Jones HW Jr, Rauramo L, Semm K, Widholm O, Wiqvist N. Helsinki statement on human *in vitro* fertilization. Ann NY Acad Sci 442:571, 1985.

Van Uem JF, Acosta AA, Swanson RJ, Mayer J, Ackerman S, Burkman LJ, Veeck LL, McDowell JS, Bernardus RE, Jones HW Jr. Male factor evaluation in *in vitro* fertilization: Norfolk experience. Fertil Steril 44:375, 1985.

Wilkes CA, Rosenwaks Z, Jones DL, Jones HW Jr. Pregnancy related to infertility diagnosis, number of attempts, and age in a program of *in vitro* fertilization. Obstet Gynecol 66:350, 1985.

Garcia JE, Jones HW Jr, Acosta AA, Andrews MC. Reconstructive pelvic operations for *in vitro* fertilization. Am J Obstet Gynecol 153:172, 1985.

Chillik CF, Acosta AA, Garcia JE, Perera S, van Uem J, Rosenwaks Z, Jones HW Jr. The role of *in vitro* fertilization in infertile patients with endometriosis. Fertil Steril 44:56, 1985.

Bernardus RE, Jones GS, Acosta AA, Garcia JE, Liu HC, Jones DL, Rosenwaks Z. The significance of the ratio in follicle-stimulating hormone and luteinizing hormone in induction of multiple follicular growth. Fertil Steril 43:373, 1985.

Jones GS, Acosta AA, Garcia JE, Rosenwaks Z. Specific effects of FSH and LH on follicular development and oocyte retrieval as determined by a program for *in vitro* fertilization. Ann NY Acad Sci 442:119, 1985.

Acosta AA, Bernardus RE, Jones GS, Garcia J, Rosenwaks Z, Simonetti S, Veeck LL, Jones D. The use of pure FSH alone or in combination for ovulation stimulation in *in vitro* fertilization. Acta Eur Fertil 16:81, 1985.

Jones GS. Use of purified gonadotropins for ovarian stimulation in IVF. Clin Obstet Gynecol 12:775, 1985.

Andrews MC, Muasher SJ, Levy DL, Jones HW Jr, Garcia JE, Rosenwaks Z, Jones GS, Acosta AA. An analysis of the obstetric outcome of 125 consecutive pregnancies conceived *in vitro* and resulting in 100 deliveries. Am J Obstet Gynecol 154:848, 1986.

Azziz R, Mulaikal RM, Migeon CJ, Jones HW Jr, Rock JA. Congenital adrenal hyperplasia: long-term results following vaginal reconstruction. Fertil Steril 46:1011, 1986.

Guzick DS, Wilkes C, Jones HW Jr. Cumulative pregnancy rates for *in vitro* fertilization. Fertil Steril 46:663, 1986.

Jones HW Jr. Ethical considerations of the new reproductive technologies. Ethics Committee of the American Fertility Society. Fertil Steril 46: Suppl 1, 1986.

Jones HW Jr. The impact of *in vitro* fertilization on the practice of gynecology and obstetrics. Int J Fertil 31:99, 1986.

Acosta AA, Andrews MC, Jones GS, Jones HW Jr, Muasher SJ, Rosenwaks Z. The indications for *in vitro* fertilization. VA Med 113:216, 1986.

Rock JA, Parmley T, Murphy AA, Jones HW Jr. Malposition of the ovary associated with uterine anomalies. Fertil Steril 45:561, 1986.

Jones GS, Muasher SJ, Rosenwaks Z, Acosta AA, Liu HC. The perimenopausal patient in *in vitro* fertilization. The use of gonadotropin-releasing hormone. Fertil Steril 46:885, 1986.

Jones GS. The physiology of menstruation and the corpus luteum function. Int J Fertil 31:143, 1986.

Lee PA, Migeon CJ, Bias WB, Jones GS. Familial hypersecretion of adrenal androgens transmitted as a dominant, non-HLA linked trait. Obstet Gynecol 69:259, 1987.

Jones GS. Reply to the Vatican "Instruction on respect for human life in its origin and on the dignity of procreation." Fertil News, Oct 1, 1987, 4.

Jones HW Jr, Schrader. The process of human fertilization: implications for moral status. Fertil Steril 48:189, 1987.

Boutteville C, Muasher SJ, Acosta AA, Jones HW Jr, Rosenwaks Z. Results of *in vitro* fertilization attempts in patients with one or two ovaries. Fertil Steril 47:821, 1987.

Romeu A, Muasher SJ, Acosta AA, Veeck LL, Diaz J, Jones GS, Jones HW Jr, Rosenwaks Z. Results of *in vitro* fertilization attempts in women 40 years of age and older: the Norfolk experience. Fertil Steril 47:130, 1987.

Liu HC, Kreiner D, Muasher SJ, Jones G, Jones HW Jr, Rosenwaks Z. β-human chorionic gonadotropin as a monitor of pregnancy outcome in *in vitro* fertilization-embryo transfer patients. Fertil Steril 50:89, 1988.

Liu HC, Jones HW Jr, Rosenwaks Z. The efficiency of human reproduction after *in vitro* fertilization and embryo transfer. Fertil Steril 49:649, 1988.

Jones HW Jr. Ethical considerations of the new reproductive technologies. Ethics Committee (1986-87) American Fertility Society. Fertil Steril 49: suppl 2, 1988.

Oehninger S, Acosta AA, Kreiner D, Muasher SJ, Jones HW Jr, Rosenwaks Z. Failure of fertilization in *in vitro* fertilization: the occult male factor. J IVF 5:181, 1988.

Brzyski RG, Muasher SJ, Droesch K, Simonetti S, Jones GS, Rosenwaks Z. Follicular atresia associated with concurrent initiation of gonadotropin-releasing hormone agonist and follicle-stimulating hormone for oocyte recruitment. Fertil Steril 50:917, 1988

Oehninger S, Acosta AA, Kreiner D, Muasher SJ, Jones HW Jr, Rosenwaks Z. *In vitro* fertilization and embryo transfer (IVF/ET): an established and successful therapy for endometriosis. JIVF 5:249, 1988.

Liu HC, Jones GS, Jones HW Jr, Rosenwaks Z. Mechanisms and factors of early pregnancy wastage in *in vitro* fertilization-embryo transfer patients. Fertil Steril 50:95, 1988.

Kreiner D, Muasher SJ, Acosta AA, Jones GS, Liu HC, Rosenwaks Z. Monitoring gonadotropin-stimulated cycles for *in vitro* fertilization and embryo transfer. JIVF 5:230, 1988.

Droesch K, Muasher SJ, Kreiner D, Jones GS, Acosta AA, Rosenwaks Z. Timing of oocyte retrieval in cycles with a spontaneous luteinizing hormone surge in a large *in vitro* fertilization program. Fertil Steril 50:451, 1988.

Muasher SJ, Oehninger S, Simonetti S, Matta J, Ellis LM, Liu HC, Jones GS, Rosenwaks Z. The value of basal and/or stimulated serum gonadotropin levels in prediction of stimulation response and *in vitro* fertilization outcome. Fertil Steril 50:298, 1988.

Oehninger S, Scott R, Muasher S, Acosta AA, Jones HW Jr, Rosenwaks Z. Effects of the severity of tubal-ovarian disease and previous tubal surgery on the results of *in vitro* fertilization and embryo transfer. Fertil Steril 51:126, 1989.

Jones GS, Muasher SJ, Liu HC. Gonadotropin stimulation protocols in the Norfolk IVFprogram-1988. J Steroid Biochem 33:823, 1989.

Jones HW Jr, Schrader C. And just what is a preembryo? Fertil Steril 52:189, 1989.

Droesch K, Muasher SJ, Brzyski RG, Jones GS, Simonetti S, Liu CH, Rosenwaks Z. Value of suppression with a gonadotropin-releasing hormone agonist prior to gonadotropin stimulation for *in vitro* fertilization. Fertil Steril 52:189, 1989.

Oehninger S, Brzyski RG, Muasher SJ, Acosta AA, Jones GS. *In vitro* fertilization and embryo transfer in patients with endometriosis: impact of a gonadotropin-releasing hormone agonist. Hum Reprod 4:541, 1989.

Hofmann GE, Toner JP, Muasher SJ, Jones GS. High-dose follicle stimulating hormone (FSH) ovarian stimulation in low-responder patients for *in vitro* fertilization. J *in vitro* Fert Embryo Trans 6:285, 1989.

Brzyski R, Jones GS, Oehninger S, Acosta AA, Kruithoff CH, Muasher SJ. Impact of leuprolide acetate on the response to follicular stimulation for *in vitro* fertilization patients with normal basal gonadotropin levels. J. *In vitro* Fert Embryo Trans 6:290, 1990.

Jones HW Jr. Cryopreservation and its problems. Fertil Steril 53:780, 1990.

Karande VC, Lester RG, Muasher SJ, Acosta AA, Jones HW Jr. Are implantation and pregnancy outcome impaired in diethylstilbestrol-exposed women after *in vitro* fertilization and embryo transfer? Fertil Steril 54:287, 1990.

Jones GS. Corpus luteum: composition and function. Fertil Steril 54:21, 1990.

Coddington C, Hassiakos DK, Harrison HC, Brzyski RG, Jones GS. Effect of a gonadotropin-releasing hormone analogue on the glucose metabolism in a diabetic patient. Gynecol Obstet Invest 30:246, 1990.

Edelstein MC, Brzyski RG, Jones GS, Simonetti S, Muasher SJ. Equivalency of human menopausal gonadotropin-releasing hormone agonist suppression. Fertil Steril 53:103, 1990.

Karande VC, Scott RT, Jones GS, Muasher SJ. Non-functional ovarian cysts do not affect ipsilateral or contralateral ovarian performance during *in vitro* fertilization. Hum Reprod 5:431, 1990.

Karande VC, Jones GS, Veeck LL, Muasher SJ. High dose follicle stimulating hormone stimulation at the onset of the menstrual cycle does not improve the *in vitro* fertilization outcome in low-responder patients. Fertil Steril 53:486, 1990.

Oehninger S, Muasher SJ, Kreiner D, Acosta AA, Jones GS. Successful ovulation induction, oocyte *in vitro* maturation and fertilization, and early embryo development in insulin-dependent diabetes mellitus. Fertil Steril 53:741, 1990.

Edelstein MC, Brzyski RG, Jones GS, Oehninger S, Sieg SM, Muasher SJ. Ovarian stimulation for *in vitro* fertilization using pure follicle-stimulating hormone agonist in high-responder patients. J *In vitro* Fertil Embryo Trans 7:172, 1990.

Hofmann GE, Scott RT, Brzyski RG, Jones HW Jr. Immunoreactive epidermal growth factor concentrations in follicular fluid obtained from *in vitro* fertilization. Fertil Steril 54:303, 1990.

Hassiakos D, Toner JP, Muasher SJ, Jones HW Jr. Implantation and pregnancy rates in relation to oestradiol and progesterone profiles in cycles with and without the use of gonadotropin-releasing hormone agonist suppression. Hum Reprod 5:1004, 1990.

Brzyski RG, Hofmann GE, Scott RT, Jones HW Jr. Effects of leuprolide acetate on follicular fluid hormone composition at oocyte retrieval for *in vitro* fertilization. Fertil Steril 54:842, 1990.

Katayama KP, Stafl A, Woodruff JD, Masukawa T, Jones HW Jr. Analysis of false negative cytology by a chromosome study. Asia Oceana J Obstet Gynecolaecol 16:85, 1990.

Muasher SJ, Kruithoff C, Simonetti S, Oehninger S, Acosta AA, Jones GS. Controlled preparation of the endometrium with exogenous steroids for the transfer of frozen-thawed pre-embryos in patients with anovulatory or irregular cycles. Hum Reprod 443-5, 1991.

Jones GS. Luteal phase defect: a review of pathophysiology. Curr Opin Obstet Gynecol 3:641, 1991.

Azziz R, Jones HW Jr, Rock JA. Androgen insensitivity syndrome: long-term results of surgical vaginal creation. J Gyn Surg 6:23, 1991

Hassiakos DK, Muasher SJ, Veeck LL, Jones HW Jr. *In vitro* fertilization: effective alternative to surgery for distal tubal occlusion. VA Med Q 118.26, 1991.

Brzyski R, Jones GS, Jones HW Jr, Oehninger S, Muasher SJ. Alterations in luteal phase progesterone and estradiol production after leuprolide acetate therapy before ovarian stimulation for *in vitro* fertilization. Fertil Steril 55:119, 1991.

Toner JP, Philput CB, Jones GS, Muasher SJ. Basal follicle-stimulating hormone level is a better predictor of *in vitro* fertilization performance than age. Fertil Steril 55:784, 1991.

Scott RT Jr, Hofmann GE, Veeck LL, Jones HW Jr, Muasher SJ. Embryo quality and pregnancy rates in patients attempting pregnancy through *in vitro* fertilization. Fertil Steril 55:426, 1991.

Toner JP, Hassiakos DK, Muasher SJ, Hsiu JG, Jones HW Jr. Endometrial receptivities after leuprolide suppression and gonadotropin stimulation: histology, steroid receptor concentrations, and implantation rates. Ann NY Acad Sci 622:220, 1991.

Jones HW Jr. Ethical and moral issues of assisted reproduction. Presented at VIIth World Congress on Human Reproduction. Ann NY Acad Sci, 626:605, 1991.

Jones HW Jr. Ethical issues in surrogate motherhood. Commentary on ACOG Committee Opinion, Number 8, November 1990. Women's Health Issues, 1:000, 1991.

Jones HW Jr. In the beginning there was Bob. Hum Reprod, Special Edition, 6:5, 1991.

Hassiakos DK, Toner JP, Jones GS, Jones HW Jr. Late-onset congenital adrenal hyperplasia in a group of hyperandrogenic women. Arch Gyn Obstet 249:165, 1991.

Jones HW Jr. Assisted reproduction. Clin Obstet Gynecol 35:749, 1992.

Seoud MA, Jones HW Jr. Indications for *in vitro* fertilization: changing trends: the Norfolk experience. Annals Acad Med 21:459, 1992.

Coddington CC, Brzyski R, Hansen KA, Corley DR, McIntyre-Seltman K, Jones HW Jr. Short-term treatment with leuprolide acetate is a successful adjunct to surgical therapy for leiomyomata uteri. Surg Gyn Obstet 175:57, 1992.

Jones HW Jr, Muasher SJ, Nusbaum R. A step toward solving some of the problems of cryopreservation. Fertil Steril 57:278, 1992.

Jones HW Jr, Toner JP. The infertile couple. New Eng J Med 329:1710, 1993.

Jones HW Jr, Veeck LL, Muasher SJ, Gibbons WE. On reporting pregnancies by ART. Fertil Steril Editor's Corner 60:759, 1993.

Jones HW Jr. Preferred protocol: controlled ovarian stimulation. J Assisted Reprod Genetics 10:461, 1993.

Khalifa E, Toner JP, Jones HW Jr. The role of abdominal metroplasty in the era of operative hysteroscopy. Surg Gyn Obstet 176:208, 1993.

Veeck LL, Amundson CH, Brothman LJ, DeScisciolo C, Maloney MK, Muasher SJ, Jones HW Jr. Significantly enhanced pregnancy rates per cycle through cryopreservation and thaw of nuclear stage oocytes. Fertil Steril 59:1202, 1993.

Jones HW Jr. The status of regulation of assisted reproductive technology in the United States. J Assist Reprod Genetics 10:331, 1993.

Kerdelhue B, Jones GS, Gordon K, Seltman H, Lenoir V, Millar RP, Williams RF, Hodgen GD. Hypothalamo-anterior pituitary gonadotropin-releasing hormone and substance-P systems during the 17 beta-estradiol-induced plasma luteinizing hormone surge in the ovariectomized female monkey. Endocrinol 132:1151, 1993.

Jones HW Jr, Edwards RG, Seidel GE. On attempts at cloning in the human. Fertil Steril, Editor's Corner, 61:423, 1994.

Toth TL, Baka SG, Veeck LL, Jones HW Jr, Muasher S, Lanzendorf SE. Fertilization and *in vitro* development of cryopreserved human prophase I oocytes. Fertil Steril 61:891, 1994.

Schoolcraft WB, Schenker T, Gee M, Jones GS, Jones HW Jr. Assisted hatching in the treatment of poor prognosis *in vitro* fertilization candidates. Fertil Steril 62:551, 1994.

Jones HW Jr, Edwards RG, Seidel GE. The best of us. Fertil Steril (Letter to the Editor) 62:893, 1994.

Damario MA, Carpenter SE, Jones HW Jr, Rock JA. Reconstruction of the external genitalia in females with bladder exstrophy. Int J Gyn Obstet 44:245, 1994.

Jones HW Jr. Reflections on the usefulness of embryo cloning. Kennedy Institute of Ethics Journal, 4:205, 1994.

Jones HW Jr. Children of choice: a doctor's perspective. Washington and Lee Law Review, 52:225, 1995.

Rock JA, Carpenter SE, Wheeless CR, Jones HW Jr. The clinical management of maldevelopment of the uterine cervix. J Pelvic Surg 1:129, 1995.

Jones HW Jr, Veeck LL, Muasher SJ. Cryopreservation: the problem of evaluation. Hum Reprod 10:2136, 1995.

Baka SG, Toth TL, Veeck LL, Jones HW Jr, Muasher SJ, Lanzendorf SE. Evaluation of the spindle apparatus of *in vitro* matured human oocytes following cryopreservation. Hum Reprod 10:1816, 1995.

Toth TL, Veeck L, Muasher SJ, Jones GS, Jones HW Jr. Factors affecting improved term pregnancy rates: the role of individualization in ovarian stimulation for *in vitro* fertilization. Presented at VIIth World Congress on IVF and Assisted Reproduction. Paris, June 1991. J Reprod Med, 1995.

Kerdelhue B, Jones GS, Gordon K, Seltman H, Lenoir V, Melik Parsadaniantz S, Williams RF, Hodgen GD. Activation of the hypothalamo-anterior pituitary corticotropin-releasing hormone, adrenocorticotropin hormone and beta-endorphin systems during the estradiol 17 beta-induced plasma LH surge in the ovariectomized monkey. J Neurosci Res 42:228, 1995.

Jones HW Jr. Twins or more. Fertil Steril, Editor's Corner, 63:701, 1995.

Jones HW Jr. Who should treat the infertile couple? Obstet Gynecol Surv, Guest Editorial 50:251, 1995.

Schoolcraft WB, Schlenker T, Jones GS, Jones HW Jr. *In vitro* fertilization in women age 40 and older: the impact of assisted hatching. J Assist Reprod Genet 12:581, 1995.

Jones HW Jr. HEFA's patient guidelines penalizes the value of embryo cryopreservation. Debate article, manuscript RO/5003, Hum Reprod 11:1364, 1996.

Jones HW Jr. Leveling the playing field. Fertil Steril, Letter to the Editor, 65:891, 1996.

Jones HW Jr. The time has come. Fertil Steril, Editors Corner, 65:1090, 1996.

Jones HWJ. On auditing ART results. Editorial, J Assist Reprod Genetics 13:4, 1996.

Jones HW Jr. Moments in the life of Patrick Steptoe. Fertil Steril 66:15, 1996.

Toth TL, Awwad JT, Veeck LL, Jones HW Jr, Muasher SJ. Suppression and flare regimens of a gonadotropin-releasing hormone agonist in women with different basal gonadotropin values in an *in vitro* fertilization program. J Reprod Med 41:321, 1996.

Kerdelhue B, Lenoir V, Kolm P, Seltman HJ, Jones HW Jr, Jones GS. ACTH, β-endorphin, substance P, and corticotrophin releasing hormone in plasma and follicular fluid in hormonally stimulated menstrual cycles for *in vitro* fertilization in the human. Hum Reprod 12:231, 1997.

Jones HW Jr, Jones D, Kolm P. Cryopreservation: a simplified method of evaluation. Hum Reprod 12:548, 1997.

Jones HW Jr, Out HJ, Hoomans EHM, Driessen SG, Bennink HJT. Cryopreservation: the practicalities of evaluation. Hum Reprod 12:1522, 1997.

Kerdelhue B, Gordon K, Williams R, Lenoir V, Fardin V, Chevalier P, Garrett C, Duval P, Kolm P, Hodgen G, Jones HW Jr, Jones GS. Stimulatory effect of a specific substance P antagonist (RPR 100893) of the human NK1 receptor on the estradiol-induced LH and FSH surges in the ovariectomized cynomolgus monkey. J Neuroscience Res 50:94-103, 1997.

Jones HW Jr. Record of the first physician to see Henrietta Lacks at the Johns Hopkins Hospital: history of the beginning of the HeLa cell line. Am J Obstet Gynecol (Suppl) 176:S227, 1997.

Jones HW Jr. The role of freezing in improving the efficiency of ART. Proceedings of evolution in ovulation induction and ART: new treatment modalities for the next millennium. Orlando, FL, March 1997.

Jones HW Jr. Training in a bygone era. Hopkins Med News, Winter 1997, 18.

Jones HW Jr. Mullerian anomalies. Hum Reprod 13:789, 1998.

Mohyi DL, Kerdelhue B, Lenoir V, Kolm P, Jones HW Jr, Jones GS. Plasma substance-P and substance-K and gonadal steroids in relation to the gonadotropin surge in normal human reproductive cycles. Clin Assisted Reprod 15:547, 1998.

Montgomery TR, Aiello F, Adelman RD, Wasylyshyn N, Andrews MC, Brazelton B, Jones GS, Jones HW Jr: The psychological status at school age of children conceived by *in vitro* fertilization. Hum Reprod 14:2162, 1999.

Develioglu OH, Hsiu JG, Nikas G, Toner JP, Oehninger S, Jones HW Jr. Endometrial estrogen and progesterone receptor and pinopode expression in stimulated cycles of oocyte donors. Fertil Steril 71:1040, 1999.

Nikas G, Develioglu OH, Toner JP, Jones HW Jr. Endometrial pinopodes indicate a shift in the window of receptivity in IVF cycles. Hum Reprod 14:787, 1999

Jones HW Jr, Crockin SL. On assisted reproduction, religion and civil law. Fertil Steril 73:447, 2000.

Kerdelhue B, Williams RF, Lenoir V, Fardin V, Kolm P, Hodgen GD, Jones GS, Scholler R, Jones HW Jr. Variations in plasma levels of substance P and effects of a specific substance P antagonist of the NK1 receptor on preovulatory LH and FSH surges and progesterone secretion in the cycling cynomolgus monkey. Reproductive Endocrinology 71:228, 2000.

Nikas G, Makrigiannakis A, Hovatta O, Jones HW Jr. Surface morphology of the human endometrium. Basic and clinical aspects. Annals of the New York Academy of Sciences 900:316, 2000.

Develioglu OH, Nikas G, Jeng-Gwang, H, Toner JP, Jones HW Jr. Detection of endometrial pinopodes by light microscopy. Fertil Steril 74:767, 2000.

Schnorr, JA, Muasher SJ, Jones HW Jr. Evaluation of the clinical efficacy of embryo cryopreservation. Elsevier Science, 169:85, 2000.

Brown SE, Mandelin E, Oehninger S, Toner JP, Seppara M, Jones HW Jr. Endometrial glycodelin-An expression in the luteal phase of ovarian cycles. Fertil Steril 74:130, 2000.

Brown, SE, Mandelin E, Oehninger S, Toner JP, Seppara M, Jones HW Jr. Histochemical localization of endometrial insulin-like growth factor binding protein-1 and –3 during the luteal phase in controlled ovarian hyperstimulation cycles: a controlled study. Fertil Steril 74:338, 2000.

Jones HW Jr. Gender reassignment and assisted reproduction. Evaluation of multiple aspects. Hum Reprod 15:987, 2000.

Adashi EY, Cohen J, Hamberger L, Jones HW Jr, deKretser DM, Lunenfeld B, Rosenwaks Z, Van Steirteghem A. Public perception of infertility and its treatment: an international study. The Bertarelli Foundation Scientific Board. Hum Reprod 15:330, 2000.

Jones HW Jr, Schnorr JA. Multiple pregnancies: a call for action. Fertil Steril 75:11, 2001.

Schnorr JA, Doviak MJ, Muasher SJ, Jones HW Jr. Impact of a cryopreservation program on the multiple pregnancy rate associated with assisted reproductive technologies. Fertil Steril 1:147-51, 2001.

Jones HW Jr. Comment: Could stem cells be derived from cryopreserved embryos? Reprod Med Online 3(2):162, 2001.

Jones HW Jr, Cohen J. IFFS surveillance 01. Fertil Steril 76(5 Suppl 2) S5-36), 2001.

Cohen J, Jones HW Jr. How to avoid multiple pregnancies in assisted reproductive technologies. Semin Reprod Med 19(3)269-78, 2001.

Jones HW Jr. The current frontiers of *in vitro* fertilization. Growth Genet Horm 18:49-53, 2002.

Jones HW Jr, Veeck LL. What is an embryo? Fertil Steril 4:658-9, 2002.

Kerdelhue B, Brown S, Lenoir V, Queenan JTJr, Jones GS,

Scholler R, Jones HW Jr. Timing of initiation of the preovulatory luteinizing hormone surge and its relationship with the circadian cortisol rhythm in the human. Neuroendocrinology 3:158-63, 2002.

Jones HW Jr. From reproductive immunology to Louise Brown. Reprod Biomed Online Suppl 1:6-8, 2002.

Jones HW Jr. Response to tribute: IVF: past and future. Reprod Bio Med Online 6(3):375-81, Article/757, 2002.

Jones HW Jr, Veeck LL. Embryos, preembryos, and stem cells: Reply of the authors. Fertil Steril 78:1355-6, 2002.

Jones HW Jr. Multiple births: how are we doing? Fertil Steril 79:17-21, 2003.

Jones HW Jr. IVF: past and future. Reprod Biomed Online 2003 Apr-May; 6(3):375-81.

Jones HW Jr. Total reproductive potential of a single cycle – to include fresh and frozen embryos? Fertil Steril 2003 Apr; 79(4): 1044.

Jones HW Jr. A big first step. Hum Reprod 2004 Nov; 19(11):2445.

Jones HW Jr. The saga of untreated congenital adrenal hyperplasia. J Pediatr Endocrinol Metab 2004 Nov; 17(11):1481-4.

Jones HW Jr. Grading a developmental continuum-now and then. Fertil Steril 2004 Dec; 82(6): 1716.

Jones HW Jr. Chorionic gonadotropin: a narrative of its identification and origin and the role of Georgeanna Seegar Jones.
Obstet Gynecol Surv 62:1-3, 2006.

Kerdelhue B, Lenoir V, Scholler R, Jones HW Jr. ACTH-cortisol
activity during the 17beta-estradiol and LH preovulatory
surges of the menstrual cycle. Neuro Endocrinol Lett Feb-Apr;
27(1-2):114-20, 2006.

Kerdelhue B, Lenoir V, Scholler R, Jones HW Jr. Substance P
plasma concentration during the LH preovulatory surge of
the menstrual cycle in the human. Neuro Endocrinol Lett Jun;
27(3):359-64, 2006.

Kerdelhue B, Andrews MC, Zhao Y, Scholler R, Jones HW Jr.
Short term changes in melatonin and cortisol serum levels af-
ter a single administration of estrogen to menopausal women.
Neuro Endocrinol Lett 2006 27(5):659-64.

Jones HW Jr, Cohen J. IFFS surveillance 07. Fertil Steril 87(4
Suppl 1):S1-67, 2007.

Jones HW Jr. Iatrogenic multiple births: a 2003 checkup. Fertil
Steril 87:453455, 2007.

Jones HW Jr. The use of controlled ovarian hyperstimulation
(COH) in clinical *in vitro* fertilization: the role of Georgeanna
Seegar Jones. Fertil Steril 90(5):e1-3, 2008,

Jones HW Jr. Luteal phase defect: the role of Georgeanna
Seegar Jones. Fertil Steril 90(5):e5-7, 2008.

Jones HW Jr, Allen BD. Strategies for designing an efficient insurance fertility benefit: a 21st century approach. Fertil Steril 91:2295-97, 2009.

Jones HW Jr, Allen BD. The future of SET (single embryo transfer) in the United States. F V & V in ObGyn, 1:111, 2010.

Jones HW Jr, Oehninger S, Bocca S, Stadtmauer L, Mayer J. Reproductive efficiency of human oocytes fertilized *in vitro*. F V & F IN Ob/Gyn 2(3):169-171, 2010

Sicignano N, Beydoun HA, Russell H, Jones Jr H, Oehninger SO. A descriptive study of asthma in young adults conceived by IVF. Reprod Biomed Online 21:812, Epub 2010.

Rock JA, Roberts CP, Jones HW Jr: Congenital anomalies of the uterine cervix: lessons from 30 cases managed clinically by a common protocol. Fertil Steril 94:1858, 2010.

Jones HW Jr, Cooke I, Kempers R, Brinsden P, Saunders D. International Federation of Fertility Societies Surveillance 2010: Preface. Fertil Steril 95:491, 2011.

Jones HW Jr: A Centenarian's Secrets for Longevity. The Yale Journal for Humanities in Medicine, March 13, 2011.

Jones HW Jr. Seven roads traveled well and seven to be traveled more. Fertil Steril 95:853, 2011.

Jones HW Jr, Allen B. The future of SET (single embryo transfer) in the United States. FV&V in OB/GYN 2:111, 2011.

Duran HE, Simsek-Duran F, Oehninger SC, Jones HW Jr,

Castora JF: The association of reproductive senescence with mitochondrial quantity, function, and DNA integrity in human oocytes at different stages of maturation. Fertil Steril 96:384, 2011.

Sarhan A, Beydoun H, Jones HW Jr, Bocca S, Oehninger S, Stadtmauer L: Gonadotrophin ovulation induction and enhancement outcomes: analysis of more than 1400 cycles. Reprod Biomed Online, 23:220, 2011.

McClamrock HD, Jones HW Jr, Adashi EY. Ovarian stimulation and intrauterine insemination at the quarter centennial: implications for the multiple births epidemic. Fertil Steril 97:802, 2012.

Adashi E, Jones HW Jr. Barrenness vanquished: the legacy of Lesley Brown. Hum Fertil 16:97, 2013.

Kulkarni AD, Jamieson DJ, Jones Jr HW, Kissin DM, Gallo MF, Macaluso M, Adashi EY. Fertility treatments and multiple births in the United States. N Engl J Med 369:2218, 2013

Simsek-Duran F, Fang L, Ford W, Swanson R, Jones HW Jr, Castora F. Age-associated metabolic and morphologic changes in mitochondria of individual mouse and hamster oocytes. PloS ONE 8:1, 2013.

Crockin SL, Ribas D, Escalante G, Nussbaum L, Jones HW Jr. Costa Rica's ban on *in vitro* fertilization deemed a human rights violation: implications for U.S. assisted reproductive technology policy and "personhood" initiatives. Fertil Steril 100:330, 2013.

Jones HW Jr. Birthplace of a breakthrough. Johns Hopkins Medicine, Fall 2013, p 17-19.

Stillman R, Richer K, Jones HW Jr. Refuting a misguided campaign against the goal of single-embryo transfer and singleton birth in assisted reproduction. Hum Reprod 10:2599, 2013.

Jones HW Jr. A tribute to Bob. Reprod Biomed Online 27:765, 2013.

Allen BD, Adashi EY, Jones HW Jr. On the cost and prevention of iatrogenic multiple pregnancies. Reprod Biomed Online. May, 2014.

Made in the USA
Middletown, DE
11 February 2022